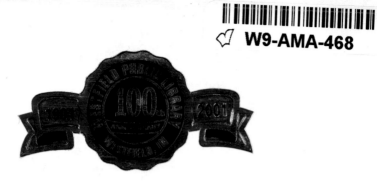
WILLOWS
on the
WINDRUSH

Also by Doris Elaine Fell
Blue Mist on the Danube

WILLOWS
on the
WINDRUSH

Sagas of a Kindred Heart

Book 2

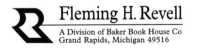

DORIS ELAINE FELL

Fleming H. Revell

A Division of Baker Book House Co
Grand Rapids, Michigan 49516

© 2000 by Doris Elaine Fell

Published by Fleming H. Revell
a division of Baker Book House Company
P.O. Box 6287, Grand Rapids, MI 49516-6287

Printed in the United States of America

Library of Congress Cataloging-in-Publication Data

Fell, Doris Elaine.
    Willows on the windrush / Doris Elaine Fell.
        p.   cm. — (Sagas of a kindred heart ; bk. 2)
      ISBN 0-8007-5732-7 (pbk.)
     1. Women chief executive officers—Fiction. 2. Inheritance and succession—Fiction. 3. Americans—England—Fiction. 4. Fathers—Death—Fiction. 5. England—Fiction. I. Title.
PS3556.E4716 W55   2000
813'.54—dc21   00-062840

For current information about all releases from Baker Book House, visit our web site:
http://www.bakerbooks.com

To
Howard and Elsie in celebration of their fiftieth anniversary

And to

Peni for her sewing room
Peter, Catherine, and Dr. Gwen Hackler for England

And especially to

Karen Steele, the author's friend and encourager

Prologue

Sydney Barrington ran along the riverbank, her bare feet leaving shallow imprints on the hard-packed sand, the chilly breeze of an early spring morning snapping at her slender legs. She jogged against the wind with strong, even strides, her somber face turned to the dusky sun, her chestnut-brown hair wind-tossed and tangled. Across the river, the melted snows of winter had turned into torrents cascading over the mountain cliff, the deluge crashing and thundering against the weather-beaten rocks in a vigorous display of power.

Sydney enjoyed this time of year in the Pacific Northwest—the closing of one season, the beginning of another. Even more, she sought comfort in these solitary moments by the river with the roaring waterfalls teasing her memory with shadowy images and stirring emotions both happy and sad. In her mind, one voice played out, time and again.

"You can't run away from responsibility, Sydney." Her father's voice. Always calling her back. *"You're a Barrington, Syd. Don't ever forget it."*

But she wasn't a Barrington. Not really. She was a Barrington in name only.

The memory broke. Sydney jogged on, pacing herself to the fast rhythm of the water as it roared and tumbled over the rocks. She sensed its frenzy, knew its rage, wanted its unstoppable freedom. She had everything and should be content, grateful.

But at the moment Sydney felt as though she had nothing of her own choosing. Her whole life had been designed

7

by the couple who had adopted her. Doting parents. Dead parents. She had inherited everything from the Barringtons, even the international defense company that Aaron Barrington had started from scratch. But she didn't want to partner with a dead father for the rest of her life. She longed for a future of her own, for a purpose not inherited.

No one seeing her now would recognize her as the elegant, successful chief executive from Barrington Enterprises—envied by some for her wealth and position, feared by others for her drive and expectations. Not even her dear, charming Randolph Iverson could guess how desperate she felt competing in a global market, pouring her life into expanding Barrington Enterprises for her dead father. It was an enormous job for anyone; Herculean for a woman barely thirty. The biggest contract of her career lay at her fingertips—the bid on two British carriers. She wanted to build them and prove to the world—to her dead father—that she could live up to the Barrington name.

As she increased her pace, savoring the freedom of running alone, another memory joggled her mind—her father holding her on his lap in his leather chair on her seventh birthday.

"And what do you want to be when you grow up, little birthday girl?"

"A wife and mommy," she said, as she cradled her baby doll in her arms. "I dropped her, Daddy, so I put a bandage on her head."

"I see that."

"Maybe I'll be a nurse and take care of little children."

He took the doll from her and dropped it nonchalantly on the floor beside his chair, then tousled Sydney's hair. "Honey, when you grow up, you won't have time for babies and dolls. Any daughter of mine is going to work with me. Now, let's go get my briefcase and I'll show you some blueprints of a fighter jet—then you'll understand how important mathematics will be to you."

She had followed him, feeling belittled and ashamed, hot tears of disappointment burning behind her eyes as they were doing now.

Above the riverbank, clumps of lantana shrubs split the winter-hardened earth in a creamy carpet of tangerine swirls. How often when she was a child her mother had helped her cut their tiny flowers for bridal bouquets for her Barbie dolls.

She ached, thinking of her mom—that gentle woman who loved Aaron Barrington—who patiently tended her garden. Before the first frost of autumn, her mother always donned boots and garden gloves to tackle her perennials. Sydney could see her now, plunging a pitchfork into the knotty roots of the lantana and splitting them in two. Then wiping her brow, she'd kneel down and replant them, patting the soil ever so gently.

"There. See how easy it is, Sydney, to dig at the tough roots and start all over again? These plants will spread and grow again in the spring and summer, and, if I live long enough, I shall enjoy the fruits of my labor."

Sydney felt like those perennials, the prongs of the pitchfork digging into her own tangled and twisted roots. The river thundered beside her, smashing into the rocks in the riverbed. Churning and spinning into whirlpools, like the whirlpools of memory sucking her into their undertow with splintered images of those last moments with her parents.

"You should go with us," Aaron Barrington had said as they stood at the boarding gate at Kennedy International. "I want you to be familiar with our foreign facilities."

"I've been abroad several times, Dad. And I know about your shipyard along the River Tyne," she teased. "I've been there."

He had poured millions into buying it. Aaron's British faux pas, his board of directors had called it. His boondoggle. Even Sydney's mother, who never questioned her husband's business moves, had considered the acquiring of an English shipyard a mistake of sizable proportion, an error in judgment.

"I'll make a go of that shipyard, Syd. Wait and see. And now—just say you'll go with us and we'll catch the next plane."

She glanced at her mother standing silently there, so short beside Aaron's towering frame. "Not this time, Dad. I'm looking into graduate courses in social work or nursing. I still want to work with children and carve out a life for myself."

Disappointment filled his dark eyes. "After all of the plans your mother and I made for you? You don't need more schooling to take over the company. I'll teach you anything you need to know."

"Your plans, Dad. Not mine."

"Honey, I thought we had an understanding. If you want to transfer to another department, just say so. But how can helping a room full of children begin to compare with building missiles and fighter jets for your country?"

For a moment she considered backing down. Then, as the boarding call was announced, he pressed his craggy cheek against hers. "You're a Barrington, Sydney. I've groomed you all your life to take over Barrington Enterprises when I'm gone."

Lightly she said, "That's a long time from now, Dad."

It was only twenty minutes before the news reached her that her parents' jet had spiraled out of the sky and plunged into the waters off Long Island . . . with no survivors.

Grief and self-recrimination engulfed her. Yet taking over the business after her father's death came with a swiftness that shocked even his closest friends. Her board of directors doubted her ability to lead, and Randolph challenged her decisions. She fought to earn their respect; the more they opposed her, the more determined she was to control the defense plants in Tennessee and California and the Barrington subdivisions abroad. And in spite of their opposition, she continued to refurbish the shipyard in England; she couldn't even give her father's botched investment away. Nor would she, not if it meant smearing his memory. But how long must she go on shoring up the loose ends of his ambitious goals before she could leave someone else in charge and move on?

Tomorrow remained an elusive vapor. No shiny, long-handled pitchfork to split the tangled roots of her father's dreams from her own. Nearing exhaustion, she stopped running and leaned against a gnarled tree to catch her breath. Her face and neck were wet with the morning dew, her clothes damp from running. Without warning, tears welled in her eyes, eyes that Randolph told her were both kind and cruel at the conference table, pensive and alluring when he was alone with her. She thrust the sleeves of her baggy sweatshirt above her elbows and brushed a twig from her faded shorts. The river rushed on, swirling, tumbling, winding around the bend in its race toward the sea, toward the open waters.

Rushing on without her.

On the other side of the world, the sleek, curving hull of the *HMS Invincible* gleamed as the aircraft carrier steamed through the azure waters of the Mediterranean. Lieutenant Commander Jonas Willoughby stood on the flight deck, thrilling to the dips and swells of the sea as he headed home to England.

Tall and sun-tanned, Jonas made an imposing figure, the wings on the sleeve of his officer's jacket well-earned. A gusty breeze whipped against his well-chiseled face. He rubbed his jaw. A stubborn one, his father called it, but then, they were cut from the same cloth—strong, disciplined men with a certain swaggering charm that appealed to women. Jonas had his dad's thick black hair and blue eyes hooded by dark brows. His high cheek bones and wide brow were more like his mother's, but again firm, well-chiseled. Mostly, with every birthday, he was his dad all over again—ambitious, driven to succeed, energetic, loyal.

As he braced his spine against the aircraft carrier's superstructure, the song in the wind kept repeating the skipper's words, over and over. "Willoughby, I have recommended you for another promotion—and a command of your own."

"I qualified then, Captain?"

His commanding officer smiled. "Must have done. Looks like you'll make commander sooner than your father did."

At thirty-four, Jonas's career was right on course. If anything, he was ahead of schedule in his climb toward the Admiralty. Nothing short of death would stop him. But as he glanced at the row of Sea Harriers, nostalgia set in. He'd flown the Royal Navy jets from the early days of his career, the aircraft as much a part of him as his arms and legs. He knew the power of the Harrier in his grasp. The daredevil exhilaration of launching from the moving deck of the *Invincible.* The triumph and risk of flying into the wind and clouds at 600 knots.

The closer he came to the ship docking in Portsmouth—to that moment when he would fly his Sea Harrier off the deck for the last time—the more reluctant he felt. His fingers lingered on his stubbly jaw. A command of his own demanded a man at peace with himself. He had learned from his father to wear a facade of calm, but his anger roiled beneath the surface, his bitterness weighing hard like rock. Three years had failed to ease his grief and that sense of unfairness at the loss of his beloved fiancée. He still carried a personal vendetta against the Irish terrorists who had murdered the woman he loved more than life itself. No matter how much he accomplished, it seemed he would never fill the void that Louise's death had left in his life.

He ducked beneath the wing of the nearest Harrier and rubbed his hand gently over the aircraft. The thought of not flying for the next eighteen months—perhaps never flying again—dug at his gut. He consoled himself with thoughts of his own ship. Not a destroyer like the *HMS Newcastle* that ran escort to the *HMS Invincible,* nor a frigate or any of the ships his father had commanded, but a 484-ton minehunter capable of operating in deep waters. Removing mines was risky, but he liked the sound of a vessel under the leadership of Commander Jonas Willoughby.

Would his father be pleased? He had a second to conjure up an image of his father's scowling gaze, dark brows puckered, slate-blue eyes scornful. "A minehunter, Jonas, not a cruiser? Wasn't flying a Harrier risky enough for you? You should have come to me. I could have put in a good word for you—"

That was his father. James Tobias Willoughby—the proud old Admiral, respected from the Admiralty down, knighted by the Queen, reduced now to glorying in the past. And Jonas, the only son, trying for a lifetime to please him.

"Sorry, Dad," he mused wryly. "I'm going to make it to the top without you pulling strings."

One

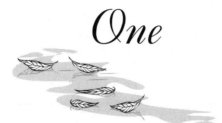

Sydney Barrington drove into her rain-drenched parking space at Barrington Enterprises and ran for the cover of the main building. At 7:00 A.M., she entered her executive suite wearing her confident public image and a stylish suit with a designer label.

"I put coffee and pastries in the conference room," her secretary said. "Your guests should be here by 8:00."

"Good." In her mind, Sydney rehearsed the details of the scheduled conference. Her father's approach to landing international contracts had been brusque. Sydney chose to use charm and feminine wiles at the conference table, along with a pot of Starbucks coffee and tempting Danish rolls. Nail this contract to build two new aircraft carriers for the Brits and it would cease being her father's company. It would be hers.

Yet the minute she stepped into the room, she was struck again by the massive dark cherry desk and the soft upholstered chair that had once been her father's throne, his powerhouse. A tan leather chair and ottoman stood by the window in the corner where her father often sat to read his reports or to reread Hemingway's *The Old Man and the Sea*.

Shrugging off the weight of her father's presence, she moved swiftly across the room and dropped her briefcase on the desk. She glanced at his photograph and saw her father's mesmerizing eyes staring back at her. "It's a big day ahead, Dad. The board of directors and Randolph are dragging their feet, but I intend to be the prime contractor on this job. I know I can take it from the design print to the blue-print to two ships at sea."

Her father had taught her everything she knew from engineering to yachting and always gave her credit as long as she did her best. Would he be pleased with her now? Yes, he would want her to win the bid on the carriers at all cost.

Through the door, she heard Randolph laughing with her secretary. Sydney busied herself sifting through her briefcase as he peeked in. "Good morning, darling," he said.

She looked up and met his gaze. "Oh, it's you, Randolph."

He tugged at his earlobe, his expression bewildered. "Should I go out and come in again?"

"Of course not. You're right on time."

Her thoughts reeled as Randy swaggered across the room to her—tall and desirable, much taller than her own five-foot-eight. As he leaned down to kiss her, she turned her head, avoiding his lips on hers.

"Why the cold shoulder, Sydney?"

"Let's get to the conference room."

"Business! That's all you think about," he said, following her. "These last few weeks, you've had our management team working double time revising the design prints and 3-D computer images. And what for?"

"So we can win that contract with the British."

He opened the door to the conference room for her. "I don't like what's happened to you since your parents died. You're power hungry one moment, the charming girl I remember the next. You're my fiancée, but this defense company keeps coming between us. It's all business. You never show your affection anymore."

"There's a time and place—"

"For me, it's always the right time. The right place."

Dear Randolph. She understood his frustration. Lately, he had grown impatient waiting for her to set their wedding date. She pulled away as he caught her hand and pressed it to his lips.

He frowned. "You're not wearing your diamond this morning."

She glanced at her finger. "Oh, I must have left it in my jewelry box." She wore it when the occasion demanded. When she remembered.

"Are you trying to impress one of those Brits?"

"Those Brits," she reminded him gently, "are all married."

"Even Nigel Tarrington?"

"Especially Nigel."

"What makes you think you'll get that contract? We're up against some stiff competition here and abroad."

Randy was undermining her again. *You don't think I can handle the job,* she thought. *But I'll prove you wrong.*

Moments later, the tweed-clad Brits filed in, no-nonsense men representing the British Defense Secretary. Peter Dykes, the retired Vice-Admiral from the Royal Navy; Graham Morrison, a barrel-chested man with a triple chin; and Nigel Tarrington, who clung to her hand long enough to bring color to her cheeks.

Her own management team came behind them—Ivy Meckerton dressed to the nines and Kleve MacMillian with a cell phone to his ear, yakking figures. Daron Emery, her best architectural engineer, with his intelligent coal-black eyes meeting hers. And Craig Edwards and Mike Spencer, two of her computer experts.

Smiles. More handshakes. The dragging of chairs and loosening of jackets as they settled around the conference table. "We trust you had a good flight over, Admiral Dykes."

"Quite comfortable, thank you, Miss Barrington."

He was brisk and to the point as he gave them an update on the plan to combine the Royal Navy and the Royal Air Force as a single air defense unit.

Randolph interrupted. "Won't that end inter-service rivalry between those units?"

"No, Iverson, it will strengthen our air fleet with pilots who can serve both on land or aboard a ship. We want those ships ready for service within the next decade." Dykes cleared his throat. "Now, let's see what you have for us."

Daron Emery unrolled the design print and spread it on the conference table for Sydney. "Gentlemen," Sydney said, "the carrier we propose for your air fleet is a 40,000-ton ship, capable of accommodating up to fifty aircraft fighters. You'll note the slant of the flight deck—"

Admiral Dykes eyed her with amusement. "Looks good."

Dykes kept that amused twinkle as they discussed the type of launchers, the speed of the ship, the cost factors—Sydney as verbal as the men.

"Admiral, your ships are much smaller than our American aircraft," Randolph interjected. "And I question your use of electric instead of nuclear power."

Sydney wanted to kick Randolph. He'd known the specs for months. If he didn't stop putting his Cincinnati foot in his mouth at every turn, she was going to order him from the conference table. She smoothed it over, saying, "Let's have a look at our 3-D computer version of the carrier."

The colored images flashed on the screen—images of pilots catapulting their Eurofighters from the flight deck. Finally she said, "Admiral, we're prepared to build those ships for you."

Dykes nodded. "But they must be built in the UK."

Sydney felt triumphant. Her dad's folly was about to pay off. "Admiral, Barrington owns a shipyard along the River Tyne."

"I personally inspected that shipyard before flying over. They were pulling a cruise ship into the dry dock when I was there. Massive place."

She gave him her warmest smile. "We're expanding so we can build those carriers for you."

"Good show, Miss Barrington. But keep in mind, we invited several defense companies to submit their bids on the new carriers." His mouth curved, half smiling. "We need your complete report within the month. We'll carry it back to England with us and personally deliver it to the project manager. By the way, Miss Barrington, I hear you have a great interest in my country."

"I was born in England—to missionary parents. They were killed in a rebel uprising in Africa shortly after my birth."

He squeezed her hand. "I'm sorry."

As the room emptied, Sydney gave Randy a thumbs-up. "So far, so good, in spite of your sour mood."

"Get involved in a long-term project over there, Syd, and you risk weakening our priorities at home."

"We'll keep the programs here right on course, and expand every chance we get. But I want Barrington to build those ships." She grinned. "Maybe I'll send you to oversee the project."

"You don't intend to put off our wedding date until after those aircraft carriers are built, do you?"

"Maybe not that long," she teased.

"Well, for our sake, I hope the contract doesn't come through. I'm afraid I'd lose you." At the open door, he turned back. "What did you mean about being born to missionary parents?"

She gazed out on the magnificent view from the windows. The day had cleared. Snow-capped Mt. Rainier peeked out from the clouds, looking like a gigantic ice-cream cone with raspberry swirls. Far in the distance lay downtown Seattle with old Smith Tower dwarfed by glass-front skyscrapers and Puget Sound crowded with ships. Without turning to face him, she said, "When my birth parents were killed, the Barringtons took me in. Gave me their name. I've been a Barrington ever since."

"You were adopted?"

Now she looked at him. "Is that a problem for you, Randy?"

"I thought the Barringtons were your birth parents."

"Aaron preferred it that way. As far as he was concerned, I *was* his daughter."

"I don't understand."

No, you never would. The right connections matter to you. It had been a matter of pride with Aaron not to mention Africa. Not to admit that she was not his own child. "You don't understand? Perhaps that's why I never told you, Randolph."

As the *HMS Invincible* plowed through the choppy waters toward the home port, Jonas Willoughby thought about Louise. Three years ago he had stood on the back of the flag deck, thinking about her.

The NATO flotilla bobbed in the waters all around him. The blades of a Lynx helicopter whirled above the captain's bridge, almost deafening the sound of footsteps coming toward him.

"Jonas Willoughby?"

Jonas had recognized the ship's chaplain and remembered thinking that the man was too young to be wearing a clerical collar, too kind to be the bearer of bad news. Before the chaplain said another word, he knew it was crushing news and felt struck by the pungent smell of the sea with a rain squall building in the west.

"Would you like to go below, Willoughby?"

"No, Chaplain. Whatever you have come to say, tell me here."

He shouted above the noise of the chopper and the shore batteries, "It's your fiancée, Willoughby."

"Louise?"

"I'm sorry, sir, but—she was killed in Ireland."

Jonas's knees had buckled. The chaplain reached out to steady him. "There must be a mistake, Chaplain. Louise and I are going to Ireland on our honeymoon."

"She traveled there alone. Her car was ambushed by Irish terrorists. . . . She didn't have a chance—"

Now, in spite of the clamoring noise on the flight deck, Jonas sensed the lift door opening. From the corner of his eye, he saw the Signal Communications Officer—walking toward him as the chaplain had done three years ago. The man stopped several yards from him. Their eyes locked.

Everything came at Jonas in slow motion. His fears. His blurred memories of Louise. Even the SCO's steps seemed curtailed by the twenty-five-mile-an-hour wind blowing on the deck.

As he reached Jonas, he said, "Lieutenant Commander Willoughby?"

"Yes." *You know that I am.*

The wind wafted the man's hair into unruly tufts. Blew his black tie out of alignment. Fluttered the message in his hand.

"This message came in marked urgent," he said.

Jonas took it, dismissing the man. As the SCO walked away, Jonas slit the security caveat with his thumbnail and frowned as he noted the return address: The Very Reverend Charles Rainford-Simms, M.A., Bishop of Monkton, The Vicarage, Stow-on-the-Woodland, The Cotswolds.

A lump threatened to cut off Jonas's windpipe. Rainford-Simms—Louise's father—the man once destined to be his father-in-law.

As he read, he remembered the methodical calm of the man's speech, his kindly eyes beneath white bushy brows—his annoying way of meddling.

Regret to advise you that things are going poorly at Broadshire Manor. Abigail Broderick is not well and the responsibility of caring for your father is a sizable task for her. Miss Broderick refuses to place him in a Navy residence.

Jonas stared blankly at the message. The Admiral ill? The man was a powerhouse of strength. Tall and athletic. Always in command. A man of iron will whose mettle showed in battle or crisis. Inflexible. Impregnable. Abigail was the only one who never bowed under his father's demanding ways.

He forced himself to go on reading.

Jonas, something must be done about the children as well.
It needs a man's hand to settle these affairs. Once before we
needed you, Jonas. . . .

What does that mean, Charles? Are you condemning me
again for delaying the wedding when my ship deployed to
the Gulf? I didn't know your daughter would travel to Ireland without me. I didn't know Louise would die there.
What did you want of me then, Reverend? To resign my
Navy commission and fly to Ireland to pick up the broken
body of my fiancée? Am I to spend the rest of my life gath-
ering up the broken threads? That was unfair, and Jonas
knew it. Louise's father was a kindhearted man, a forgiving
man.

Jonas's fist doubled as he read of the growing problems at
the manor. Go home to a sick father, to a dwindling staff?
It seemed clear that Rainford-Simms once again did not
comprehend Jonas's commitment to the Royal Navy.

Don't you understand, Charles? A naval officer doesn't sacri-
fice his career for personal difficulties.

If the Admiral and the manor were too much for Abigail,
he would sell the place. Of what value was the property to
Jonas? It was riddled with memories of Louise and what
might have been.

He stood rigid as though he were standing in front of the
Admiral and receiving a dressing-down. *Stand easy*, he told
himself. *It's just Rainford-Simms blowing dust into a storm cloud.*
A few ship-to-shore messages and matters could be settled.

But Jonas felt his career hurtling to a standstill, and for
what? Give up his promotion to commander because the
admiral needed him? Not likely. The distance that separated
the Admiral and himself was more than nautical miles. He
admired the old man, but they stayed constantly at odds. If

Jonas gave in and went home, what would happen to his resolve to keep to his own course?

As he balanced against the swaying ship, Louise and his father meshed in his thinking. He'd give the world to have one more chance to tell Louise how much he loved her— to tell her how sorry he was for the way she died. Now was he man enough to make peace with his father before time ran out—to work up the courage to tell him how much he had idolized him all these years?

Charles's message concluded with,

Perhaps coming back to the Cotswolds would comfort you, son, as it did me. At last, I have come to terms with Louise's absence and have become a man of peace, a man of joy by staying here. My daughter was dear to me. I daresay your whole life and mine were centered in her. And you, son— three years of silence from you. Louise would want our friendship to go on. I know that you miss her dreadfully, as I do. I think of her always . . .

Jonas smashed the message into his palm.
Miss her? He still felt dead inside without her.

Twenty minutes later Jock Hollinsworth crossed the deck toward the spot where Jonas stood. He hesitated, not wanting to break into his squadron commander's solace. They'd been friends since Dartmouth, had earned their wings for fixed aircraft together. Jock had flown wingman for Jonas on more than one dangerous sortie in the Balkans and over Kosovo. He took the remaining strides and cuffed Jonas's shoulder.

"I expected to find you up here with your golf club, spinning a golf ball off the deck into the depths of the sea."

Jonas smiled. "Not after the last sounding rebuke. You know the rules. No ditching of any gash or garbage over the sides. Nothing hazardous to the aircraft. Including golf balls."

The skipper's standing rebuke was in Jonas's file, one of the few black marks there. These days Jonas kept to jogging and a regimen of exercise that kept his body trim and fit.

"The captain should ban bagpipes on board too."

"I don't practice often," Jonas defended.

"It has to be that Scottish blood in you."

"My mother's side. You know I'm British born, but I'm proud of my Scottish heritage. So I'll take the bagpipes with me when I leave, but I'll miss flying with you when I take command of my own ship. With any luck, I'll be on patrol off Northern Ireland."

Jock's jaw tightened. "Let the government settle your problems with the IRA. Whoever set off the bomb that killed Louise didn't know her. She was just an innocent traveler."

"I should have been with her."

"It didn't work out that way. Look, old man, just stay out of the Irish waters. You've earned the promotion. You've given the Royal Navy a good return of service. Peace-keeping duties in the Adriatic. Patrolling the Scandinavian waters and the oil fields of the North Sea. Bosnia. Kosovo. Jonas, you're a climber. All I ever wanted to do was fly."

"It's been a good life—belonging to Her Majesty's Navy."

"Right on. The best of both worlds. Access to every club on land. Unbeatable camaraderie at sea. But I worry about you. Anger at the IRA could ruin your career. Focus on your future. You'll be in the Admiralty before we know it. And I count on our still being friends when you reach it."

"That goes without saying, Jock."

As the crimson of a burnished sunset glowed on the horizon, Jonas pulled the bishop's crumpled message from his pocket and thrust it at Jock. "Here. Read this. I've got problems."

After reading, Jock sputtered, "Ignore this. I don't think the Admiral is your responsibility."

"He's my father, Jock."

"Somebody should have reminded him of that long ago."

"I just had difficulty pleasing him."

"No wonder, with a distinguished career like James Tobias Willoughby's—that's like filling size twenty clodhoppers."

Jonas shook his head. "Dad earned every promotion."

"No argument there. Your dad's really switched on when it comes to the Royal Navy, so let the Navy take care of him. They have rest centers in Portsmouth, don't they?" Jock gave the paper a twist of his own. "Have Abigail Broderick look into one." He gripped Jonas's shoulder. "This Rainford-Simms; he's not—?"

Jonas's eyes turned a frosty blue. "Yes. He's Louise's father."

"Sorry, old man—but my advice still stands. Let the Navy take care of the Admiral. You deserve a command of your own."

Days later, after months' deployment, the *HMS Invincible* moved into home waters on a steady course toward the south coast of England. The captain ordered the Fleet Air Arm to follow standard procedure. The Sea Harriers were to leave the ship first; the Sea King helicopters would follow.

Jonas looked around the quarters he had shared with Jock and packed the last of his toiletries into his kit. Then he picked up Louise's photograph, dusted it with his sleeve, and stared at her lovely face. "Like I promised you, Louise, I'm finally coming home."

He secured the picture snugly between his shirts and underwear and zipped his kit bag. As he squared his tie, he consoled himself that he was not leaving Her Majesty's Service—just transferring temporarily to Northwood Headquarters near London.

When he opened the door, Jock was just coming back from the wardroom. "Time to fly, Jonas."

Jonas looked at his friend's nubby skin, red from the sun, and at the ginger freckles across his nose and chin. Even his scalp looked sunburned beneath the cropped sandalwood hair. He met Jock's gaze with a crooked smile. "I guess this is it?"

"Keep in touch. My wife has some pretty young debutantes in London that she wants you to meet."

"Tell her I need more time."

"You have to get on with your life."

"The IRA took my life from me when they killed Louise." He could not imagine filling the photo frame with someone else's picture, let alone allowing himself to care deeply for another woman. "No one else could take her place."

As they reached the flight deck, Jonas shaded his eyes and stared into the clouds. "I'll miss flying the Harrier."

"Sure you will—until you command your own ship. It will be Commander Willoughby the next time we meet. I envy you."

He shouted above the bedlam. "Jock—I turned the command down. My transfer to Northwood came through two days ago."

Anger turned Jock's face scarlet. "You can't be serious—turning down your first command for a landlocked job? That won't set well in your record. I dare say you made the wrong decision."

"Once things are settled at home, I'll be back."

"But not in command of your own minesweeper?"

"No. But maybe back in command of my own life."

They shook hands. "I'm the last one off this time. Captain's orders. I want to watch the rest of the squadron leave the flight deck one more time. We've had orders to lay over in the area until the ship docks. After that, we'll meet up in Scotland."

"Will do. I'm not lingering around Scotland long. My wife's picking me up. I'm taking a forty-two-day leave. I plan to build up my flying hours in my uncle's Learjet. You remember Rodney Christopher, don't you? Uncle Rodney keeps urging me to give up the Royal Navy and go full-time with him."

"Doing what?"

"Flying his company plane. He does country hops. Sweden. Finland. Italy. Germany. He'd pay well. But don't worry, Jonas, I have no intention of leaving the Service. I want to be around when those new carriers are commissioned."

"By then age will ground us both."

"I know. I'll be too old to fly the new planes, but at least I'd like to be on board watching the younger jocks take off."

"Don't spend too much time in that Learjet."

With a wicked grin, Jock said, "I'm spending most of my leave with my wife. We're going away. Just the two of us. We've been talking about starting a family—"

Jonas thumped Jock's arm. "Then you won't miss me."

As Jonas flew above Portsmouth harbor, the city greeted the *HMS Invincible* with a rousing welcome. The waving and cheering swept him back to the day Louise met his ship for the first time. The piping of music had been interrupted by the order, "Attention, ship's company. All off-watch personnel to man the portside. That is all."

He had slipped up beside Louise as she searched the faces of the men lined up on board the ship. Searching for him. He put his arms around her and kissed her.

"Jonas, you are supposed to be on that ship," she had cried.

"Honey, it's standard procedure for pilots to fly off hours before the ship reaches harbor."

"Jonas Willoughby, why didn't you warn me?"

"I wanted to surprise you."

It was then that he realized how much he loved her—this lovely, sensitive creature—who had loved him back. He had been smitten by her beauty, her warmth and laughter when she was with him. He liked to remember her that way— that day. The day he proposed.

In the three years since her death, she had become a veiled mist, real only in his thoughts and dreams, always out of grasp. He wondered now with the exhilarating thrust of the Harrier in his control whether she would have ever adapted to his long months at sea, to his love of the Royal Navy that all too often surpassed even his commitment to her.

The demands of flying drew him back. Below him, the pearl blue of the sky reflected in the water as another warship slipped from the jetty and moved out into the channel. An American supercarrier lay anchored off the Spithead, the ship too big for Portsmouth harbor. Cruisers lay berthed at the docks, frigates and tankers by the Middle Wall. And in its permanent location stood Lord Nelson's old flagship, the *HMS Victory*.

The *Invincible* lay berthed at the South Railway Jetty now, her flight deck empty of planes. The White Ensign flew at her stern, the Union Jack on the bow. Jonas saluted with the tip of his fingers and fought the miserable lump in his throat. From the action below he knew that people were cheering. He gave the order and the squadron of Sea Harriers did another flypast, over the ship. The Sea Kings flew in formation behind them. Now some of the waving was directed toward them.

Moments later, the pilots began the return journey to their Naval Air Stations—the helicopters to their base in Cornwall and Jonas's squadron to northern Scotland. Jonas broke formation and flew once more over the carrier. He dipped his wing in salute to his ship—and to the memory of the girl who would never be on dock waiting for him again. Then he turned north toward Scotland to follow his squadron home, his future uncertain.

Two

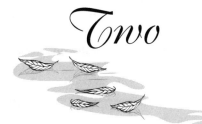

Spring bathed itself in a glorious rainbow of pastel colors, scenting the sleepy hamlet of Stow-on-the-Woodland with wild thyme and the delicate fragrance of herbs and roses. Abigail Broderick stared out the mullion windows at Broadshire Manor, down on a quiet, unpretentious village. She had spent most of her lifetime tucked away in Gloucestershire in this English village that was rooted in the past, untouched by the passing of time.

She knew little of fame or fortune, yet her years of living in someone else's magnificent manor had made her confident, wiser. A woman of stately carriage with silver gray hair and a softly curving mouth, she had always been much loved in the village.

Her distant past remained hidden, forgotten by those who knew her best. Secrets were stowed away in the chambers of her own heart and mind, laid there like an unfinished quilt in a hope chest. Her past awakened from time to time by little things—the ringing of the church bell at St. Michael's, the rain pelting on her bedroom window, the bubbling flow of the River Windrush. And recently, by the sight of Jonas lifting his ill father in his arms and carrying him to the chair by the window. But always when those unhappy memories of the past flashed back, they were overshadowed by an arc of forgiveness. Perhaps, as her dearest friend Griselda Quigley said, it was part of growing old—this being at peace, this accepting what you could not change and garnering up instead treasures for the life that lay ahead.

These days Abigail took pleasure in her walled garden and the plump buds of her blue delphiniums or the wood lilies that lazed beneath the oak. Mostly, as she had done over the years, she found her greatest joy in the children. She shared their longing for freedom—theirs from books and schoolmasters, hers from pain and the demands of growing older. As if to mock her, a sharp jolt ran through her chest, shortening her breath. There was no time to step across the room to the safety of her chair. She groped for her medicine bottle in her skirt pocket and placed a tiny tablet under her tongue, praying that the lightheadedness would not come this time. Gratefully, with a sudden flush, the vessels opened and the pain trickled away.

Shortly, she must call the children in for dinner. Mrs. Quigley expected them at the table on time. Abigail pressed her forehead against the window casing, waiting for her strength to return. She expected to see Jonas pushing the wheelbarrow toward the shed, his black-and-white collie at his heels and young Gregor tracking in Jonas's footsteps over the high rolling wolds. But Jonas was nowhere to be seen. Dear Jonas! Even in his few weeks back in the village, a persistent scowl had wedged between his brows. But she made no effort to send him away. Found no courage to tell him she could manage the manor alone.

Absently, she placed the medicine bottle on the dresser and selected a sweater from the top drawer. Stepping gracefully, as she always did, she made her way down the curving stairwell with her hand firmly on the rail. Then, plodding slowly down the entry hall, she felt her flagging heart set the pace, her pulse so irregular that she could not count the drumbeat of her own heart.

Taking the next step over the parquetry floor, she felt another age-old pain deepen inside her as she thought of Sir James Willoughby and the four young refugee children still in her care. The thought of permanently closing the doors of Broadshire Manor filled her with foreboding.

Above her a glittering chandelier hung from the coved ceiling, casting dancing shadows on the lovely portrait of Lady Helen Willoughby. Abigail remembered her own arrival as a young woman and the courage it took to grip the knocker seeking employment again. The door had been opened, not by Lady Helen, but by the lord of the manor—a tall naval officer with smashing good looks, thick black hair, and heavy-lidded, dark blue eyes that questioned her arrival.

The tower bell of St. Michael's chimed the hour, its sonorous tone slicing into her thoughts. Her chest constricted with pain as she hurried the last few steps and swung back the massive door as she always did at sunset to make certain all her children were in.

The sloping hills of the Cotswolds cast their golden glow in the fading twilight in a sky still lit with a murmur of blue. The air smelled sweet with the flowering shrubs and the wild English primroses that thrived against the drystone wall. It was all there—the peaceful, pastoral setting of a lifetime spreading out before her, even the small thatched cottage where she had been born. But the manor was her place of residence now—a massive three-story house built during the wool trade by Lady Willoughby's family, a commanding structure that dwarfed the rest of the village. Above the gold and emerald fields, fleecy clouds drifted toward eventide as one by one the village children were called in for the supper hour and bedtime.

Since Lady Willoughby's death, Abigail had reveled in running the manor for the Admiral and filling it with children who knew nothing of the value of the bronze statues or the art treasures in the library. Over the years, to the horror of the staff, Abigail's refugee children raced up and down the grand curving staircase and slid down the bronzed balustrade. They hid behind the brocade curtains and shouted in the lavish ballroom where Lady Willoughby's ancient pedestal clock still ticked.

A rustle in the bush at the foot of the stone steps caught her attention. "Gregor?" she called.

The nine-year-old peeked out, a lopsided grin filling his face. "Yes, Miss Abigail."

"So there you are. Have you been collecting bugs and crickets again to scare the girls?"

He stood pigeon-toed, a momentary stance with the scuffed toes of his shoes turned in, and the inside pockets of his trousers turned out. "Don't have nothing, Miss Abigail."

"Anything," she corrected.

He brushed his hands free. "See? Nothing."

"Then have you been with Jonas again?"

He nodded, his lustrous black eyes sparkling, his voice high-pitched, excited. "I helped him take the sheep in."

She could not fault him for this; he felt safe with Jonas. Still, she said, "Jonas should have sent you home sooner."

"But we saw a stranger down by the river."

She allowed her eyes to graze past the thicket of woods east of the manor to the silhouette of the bridge where so many of her children had crossed over, where so few of them ever came back.

"I see no one, Gregor."

"Me and Jonas saw him."

"Jonas and I," she corrected.

He twisted the pockets of his corduroys. "I thought my papa had come back."

Her heart lurched. "Someday, Gregor. Someday, perhaps."

But we are never going to find him, she thought. Not after months of scouring desolate towns and crowded refugee camps filled with tatter-ragged families, or checking the International Red Cross lists of missing names. No, she sensed in her heart that Gregor's village was swallowed up in rubble—his family with it.

"Gregor, you'd best come in and wash up. Your supper is getting cold. Griselda made your favorite—hot dumpling stew."

His muddy sneakers squeaked as he raced up the steps. She cupped his smudged cheek before he could dart past her. "Did you play in the water, Gregor?"

"I was chasing Jonas's dog."

The black-and-white collie that comforted him. "You know you must not stay out when it's getting dark," she scolded softly.

"I'm not afraid with Jonas."

Would he be afraid if he knew that Jonas had flown sorties over Kosovo? Dropped missiles, perhaps on the village where Gregor once lived. Or would Jonas still be Gregor's hero? The boy thrilled with tales of Jonas launching his Sea Harrier off the deck of the *HMS Invincible* on a mission to destroy. She shuddered even now at the thought of his plane armed with deadly Amraam missiles patrolling the skies over Yugoslavia. Trembled at the thought of Jonas's plane coming back from combat and dropping through the night clouds onto the carrier's sleek deck. It seemed to Abigail that the boy and the man had been destined to meet—that roaming the Cotswold hills together with the black-and-white collie between them offered healing to them both.

Gregor was much like Jonas had been as a boy. An intelligent child, bent on his own way. At times angelic or curious. Sometimes a rogue, straying beyond the manor to fish along the river or dawdle on the hills. She feared what would happen when Jonas went back to sea duty and the boy was left to wander alone.

"Gregor, give Griselda your wet shoes. She'll make certain they're dry by morning."

She watched him go—her boy with those solemn dark eyes and fragile smile that had tugged at her heart the day she first saw him at the refugee camp. Gaunt. Frightened. Hungry. At the peak of the conflict, she had salvaged him from the tinderbox in Kosovo—snatched him from the arms of an Albanian guerrilla in a tattered surplus uniform who held him out to her.

"There's no one else left in his village," the man had said.

No one else left. Odd. Gregor, of all the children, feared darkness, and yet he was always the last one in.

She lingered at the door, listening for the sound of Jonas's bagpipes. She heard only the bubbling gurgle of the Windrush as it flowed beneath the old stone bridge. The river was as dear and familiar to her as the bleating sheep in the meadows, or tea and crumpets with Jonas in the late afternoon; it was as comforting as sitting with Sir James and patting his wrinkled hand while he rambled on about matters aged as the hills around them.

She glanced at the cottage on the edge of the property and saw the light in Jonas's window flicker on, saw the plumes of smoke rise from his chimney. She loved Jonas as her own son, but was it fair to let him take on the burden of the manor and the children and Sir James? He should be finding a life's companion, settling down to his own happiness. Or going back on sea duty as a pilot—to the career he loved.

From where she stood—reluctant to close out another day—she searched the darkness again. This time Abigail saw someone crossing over the bridge—a lanky man with one child sheltered in his arms and another by his side. They came stealthily now in the shadows of the evening, making their way toward the manor.

The gate squeaked as the man thrust it open. His presence set Abigail's heart to racing erratically. She tugged her sweater against her chest. He lifted his bristly face as he neared the steps, his eyes hollow even in the semi-darkness. His shoulders hunched forward under the weight of the child in his arms.

"Abigail, I was afraid you would shut the door before we could reach you."

She recognized him now—a young man who had once lived in her home. A bleak twig of a man now.

"Conon O'Reilly," she murmured. "You've come back."

"And I brought my children with me."

The boy in his arms was three at most; the little girl clutching at his side not much older.

"Conon, the last I heard, you were hiding out in Ireland."

"Then am I not welcome, Abigail?" He climbed the steps to stand level with her. "I've come in peace. Don't turn us away."

She touched his rough cheek and felt the jagged scar that ran the length of his jaw. He was still her boy, her troubled Irish boy. She tried to remember the innocent child that he had once been, but gazing up into his hollow, empty eyes, she knew a young Irish terrorist, a revolutionary, stared back at her.

Three

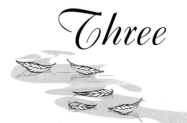

Abigail's mind was awash with memories. Recollections of a boy running away from the manor fourteen years ago. And the images of headlines since then. Belfast. Northern Ireland. Sinn Fein. The Good Friday Agreement. IRA bombings in Omagh. The failure to decommission—the failure to lay down arms.

She shuddered. "Were you followed here, Conon?"

"Would it matter?"

"It might if anyone comes looking for you."

"By then, I should be some distance from here. Please, Abigail, may we come in? The children are exhausted."

"Was it wise for you to come back?" she whispered.

"Aren't you the one who always keeps the door open until all of your children are in?"

She bit her lip, and, with another cautious glance into the darkness, stepped back to make room for them to cross the threshold. She could see Conon clearly now as he bolted the door and wedged his back firmly against it. He looked older than his twenty-nine years. A week's stubble of beard marred his once handsome face. Wiry red brows failed to hide his shifty gaze. His eyes swept the room, lingering briefly on the windows that looked out on the fountain.

He was always in trouble as a boy, the outcast of the Broderick household. Conon, her firebrand, the malcontent among the other children, defending Northern Ireland's conflict with Britain. Back then, he seemed like a stormy petrel in flight, a child constantly at war with himself. A man still at war.

When Conon focused his attention on her again, his anguished expression was bedeviled, tormented, out of reach. This troubled child who had grown into a troubled man had obviously hit upon hard times. His worn tweed jacket and dark corduroys were not nearly warm enough for a man on the run. Abigail's faith in the God who looked over the woodlands wavered, yet she felt certain Conon had not come back to harm her. Whatever his sins or misdoings—and she feared they could be legion—he had taken great risks to bring his children to her. They had his red hair, the girl his intense green eyes, wide with mistrust.

"Are you alone, Abigail?"

"I never was alone. This is a big house, remember? Most of the old servants are gone, but three of the staff stayed on. Boris and my housekeeper are still with me. You remember them." She smiled thinly. "Griselda came back after you left. I couldn't run the place without her."

"You can't keep a mansion like this with three servants."

"We manage. Part of the upper floors and the east and south wings are closed off. Opened only for dusting."

"It's not like when I was a boy, is it?"

"Nor like the glory days when Lady Willoughby was alive."

"There's no one else here?"

Her heart raced. She would not mention Jonas, but she said, "The Admiral lives here now. He's old and ill, and I still have four young refugee children. The oldest is nine—a boy from Kosovo. Two are from the Gulf War, one from Bosnia."

"Then you won't mind two from Ireland?"

She glanced at the O'Reilly children again. Neither child was dressed warmly enough for the evening chill. The girl looked rumpled and mussed, her sweater shaggy. The boy's thin legs were bare, his tousled hair partly covered by a brown cap. As sleepy as he was, he clung to a toy truck. She reached out and linked her fingers with the sleeping child.

"Conon, when did your children eat last?"

"This morning. We had some hard rolls and milk."

"That was hours ago."

"We had to keep going. I had to time our arrival toward dark. I couldn't risk anyone recognizing me in Bourton-on-the-Water."

As she took a step, intending to pull the tapestry cord, he gripped her wrist. "What are you doing?"

"I was going to ring for Griselda. I want her to feed and bathe the children."

"Not yet. Not until we settle something."

She pulled free and rubbed her wrist. Tentacles of fear knotted her stomach. Long ago he had threatened to get even with Jonas over boyish quarrels. "Settle what, Conon?"

"I want you to raise Danny and Keeley for me. Will you?" Even his voice was toneless, without hope, measured by defeat, his life empty except for these children.

"Broadshire has never been a place for fugitives. I won't let it be now." She shook her head. "Look at me. Don't you understand? My work at Broadshire Manor is drawing to a close. I've grown old since you went away. Surely you've noticed."

He blew a kiss across Danny's ear. "You've never turned a child away before, Abigail."

"But I know who you are now—what you stand for."

"You have always known what I stood for."

She ran her hand nervously across her chest. "I hoped you would change. That you would want peace."

He looked perplexed. "I do. Peace for Ireland."

Outside a tree branch scraped against the windowpane. His gaze darted from window to window and then down the long, empty corridor. He jabbed his hand into his bulging pocket, his eyes wild.

"No firearms, Conon. It's just the evening wind. Don't you remember how it would stir as darkness set in?"

"All I remember is how dark it used to be."

38

"What kind of trouble are you in that you want to leave your children behind?"

He rubbed his bristled chin against his son's cheek. Danny awakened with a start, his enormous eyes too large for the narrow ragamuffin face. Seeing his father, his eyelids drooped again.

"Trouble, you call it. Can't you even guess, Abigail?"

"I don't even know why you went away fourteen years ago."

"I wanted my children to grow up to love Ireland."

Her throat constricted. "That's what I wanted for you—to be proud of your country, to help bring peace to Northern Ireland."

"That's why I went away—why my people recruited me."

"You were only a boy then."

"Man enough to side with the IRA. It was my duty."

A sharp pain caught her breath. She walked unsteadily to the marble bench and sank down onto it. He went and sat beside her, balancing his son on his knee. Keeley squirmed against him.

"Abigail, what is it?"

The pain tracked along her jawbone. She grappled in her skirt pocket, but the medicine bottle was not there. And then she recalled with a certainty that she had left her pills on the dresser top when she went to call the children in. She pressed her hand against her chest. "I'm not well. My heart is giving out. Any excitement sets it to fluttering."

"Should I call Mrs. Quigley?"

"No, she worries enough about me."

She sat motionless, allowing her erratic heartbeat to ease. Sensing Keeley's alarm, she said, "I'll be all right, child."

"It's just—I've upset her," Conon said.

His troubled gaze turned to the fountain outside the window where two carefree children were carved in marble. Water poured from the pitcher in the girl's hand and the ring jets behind her sent geysers of water back into the pool.

The changing patterns in the water spout punctuated their silence with a symphony of their own.

He broke their silence, saying, "I remember sitting here with you as a boy the night before I ran away. I didn't mean to disappoint you. I always felt safe with you."

"Then why did you go away?"

His gaze shifted back to her. "I told you—to fight for my country."

He covered his son's ears, slipping from terrorist to father in that simple act of gentleness. "I wanted peace for Ireland. You must believe me."

"Peace? What about the Omagh incident? And those senseless killings? I hear you were involved."

"Please, Abigail. Not here, not in front of the children." His arm tightened around his son. "My children are not at war, Abigail. We have nowhere to go. Will you take them?"

The tired lines around his eyes deepened. "Let me rest a few days too? I could watch over you."

She patted his hand. "No, dear boy. I know this was your home once. Your running away never changed that. But I can't let you stay." She wished with all her heart that Conon could be a boy again. That she didn't have to send him away. "You see, there's something I haven't told you. Jonas came back a few weeks ago to settle the affairs at Broadshire Manor. He's staying out in the cottage, but he comes toward midnight to take care of his father."

He groaned. "So Jonas is back at the manor. No wonder you're afraid of my being here." His mouth twisted. "You were always forced to choose between us."

"That's not true, Conon." But she knew that it was.

At the sound of footsteps in the corridor, they whirled around on the bench, and stood. Abigail felt a flood of relief when her housekeeper stepped from the shadows.

"It's all right, Conon. It's Mrs. Quigley."

"Abigail, you promised to have supper with the—" Surprise lit Griselda's tired gray eyes. "So *you're* back! And what do we have here?"

"Two hungry children," Conon told her.

"Well, you know your way to the kitchen, Conon O'Reilly."

"So you do remember me?"

Her thick gray brows twitched. "Couldn't forget the likes of you. You used to steal biscuits hot from the oven. Yours?" she asked, nodding at the children.

Keeley shrank against her father. "Yes, this is my daughter, Keeley. And this boy in my arms is Danny."

Her gaze locked on Conon. "I trust Commander Willoughby doesn't know you're here. You best know now—Jonas has strong feelings about what you've been doing."

"A man has a right to defend his own country. But I'm not looking for trouble here, Mrs. Quigley. I'm just trying to find a safe place for my children."

Griselda touched Danny's cheek with her work-reddened hand. "The boy's feverish," she accused.

"And hungry, like I said."

"There's plenty of dumplings. For you too if you want some."

Abigail shook her head. "Conon and I will have supper in the drawing room and then he must leave. Ask Boris or Lucas if they can see Conon safely out of the village and on his way to Bourton-on-the-Water."

"Never mind, Abigail. I know my own way out of town."

"Best that way," Griselda agreed. "Besides, Lucas hasn't come in for dinner yet." The scowl on Griselda's wrinkled face deepened. "And what if Jonas asks after you, Abigail, while you and Mr. O'Reilly are in the drawing room?"

"Tell him I'm resting. I'll see him in the morning."

Griselda's eyes narrowed with disapproval. "It won't be good telling him an untruth."

"But it would be a disaster for Jonas and Conon to meet."

Griselda rubbed the back of her hand with her thumb. "The Reverend Rainford-Simms called. Should I tell him that you'll ring him back tomorrow too?"

"Was it urgent?"

"The usual. He's distressed about Jonas not dropping in. Says there's no need for them not to be friends."

Abigail shot a guarded glance toward Conon. Only the curl of his lip suggested curiosity. "Yes, Griselda, tell the reverend I'll ring back tomorrow, would you?"

Griselda shrugged irritably. Then, as she had done over the years, she took charge of the children. She lifted Danny from Conon's arms and cradled him. "He's light as a hot biscuit."

She reached out for Keeley's hand. "It's time to get you two washed up and fed."

Keeley clung to Conon. "Don't leave me, Daddy."

As he brushed back shocks of red hair from her forehead, the corners of his mouth sagged. "Your papa lived here as a boy."

Keeley's lips puckered. "I don't want to stay here."

Conon stood rock-still, sweat beading his brow. "Go with Mrs. Quigley. You'll be safe here. She will give you and Danny some supper. Later—later we can talk about it."

Griselda started toward the kitchen with a firm grip on Keeley's hand. As the child wailed, Griselda glanced back at Abigail. "Will the children be staying with us?"

"At least for the night."

Strands of wiry gray hair slipped loose as she shook her head. "That's what you always say. Should they sleep on the second floor with the other children?"

"No. Not tonight." She avoided Conon's eyes. "After their supper, you must take them to the safety of the west wing."

Danny's head bobbed sleepily against Griselda's massive bosom. "But the west wing is Sir James's quarters."

"The Admiral will not mind, nor will he remember."

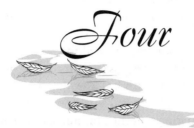

Four

Conon's iron mask dropped as a closed door silenced Keeley's sobs. Abigail put her hand on his arm. "Conon, you are breaking Keeley's heart."

"There's no other way to save her life and Danny's."

"Can't you take your children back to their mother?"

His voice rang with bitterness. "My wife, Rorie, was killed in the crossfire in Northern Ireland. If I had only known she was shopping at the market in Omagh—but I was told that the car bombing was just meant for a warning. That no one would be hurt."

"A warning? The Omagh incident broke the peace agreement. It killed twenty-eight innocent people and injured many more." *Twenty-nine dead,* if she counted Rorie.

"Believe me. We didn't intend for anyone to die there."

"How can you erase Omagh from your conscience? The peace won't work if any of you keep fighting. All they want is for you to lay down arms—"

He was incensed. "Give in, you mean? Sell out. Throw away everything we fought for. What we died for."

She tried to rest her hand on his wrist. He jerked free. "I belong to a fractional group—the real IRA," he boasted. "Omagh is only a taste of what will happen if they try to defeat us."

"That would ruin peace for everyone. It has become your personal war, hasn't it? Your battle against society. Do the children know about their mother?"

"They know she is dead. Keeley was with Rorie the day she died. Not a good memory for any child." The nerve along his jaw throbbed. "I never intended to bring any children into the world. Then Rorie became pregnant with Keeley. We married right after she was born." His voice mellowed. "And then our son came along."

He massaged his temples, his gaze steady. "Rorie was born in Dublin, as proud an Irish lass as ever was. Good-looking farm girl. Soft spoken. She was a wonderful mother, but you must never tell anyone that the children came from Ireland."

She felt a faint smile touch her lips. "You don't think people will recognize their Irish brogue? Jonas will figure it out when he sees the children. Your son looks like you."

"A rough sentence for any child." He turned his gaunt face to Abigail. "You used to keep pictures of all of your children in the drawing room. Am I still there?"

She hesitated. "No. Jonas took your picture down three years ago after one of the IRA bombings."

"Why? The IRA never hurt Jonas."

"You're wrong. Jonas suffered a great loss in one of your bombings—another isolated incident where a friend of his was killed when she turned off on the wrong road. She wasn't a threat to the IRA. But it didn't matter. They bombed her car anyway."

Conon went deathly pale. "Did it happen near Belfast?"

"Does it make a difference? Nothing can change the fact that she's gone. Come, I want you to eat before you leave."

She linked her arm in his to steady herself as they walked into the library. He flicked on the light as they entered and for a long time stood looking at the photographs of the children who had passed through the manor. "When I was a boy, we could only come in here and to the gallery on guided tours."

She laughed. "Was I that strict?"

"You were just trying to preserve the Willoughby collection. We left enough imprints on the rest of the house— sliding down the balustrade, scratching the ancient furniture, and ruining the flower beds in our scuffles."

Lightly she asked, "Do you remember carving your initials C.O.W. on the family crest? Your initials are still there. I know the C.O. stands for Conon O'Reilly. But why the W?" she asked.

"Can't you guess? It was for Willoughby. I wanted to belong to someone—to have a brother like Jonas. But why did you leave my initials out on the gate?"

"They were all I had left to remind me of you."

He picked at a loose thread on his jacket. "My photo used to hang here, right beside Jonas. Tell me, why did Jonas resign his Navy commission to come back to the Cotswolds?"

"He didn't, but he had to forgo a command of his own when he transferred to Fleet Headquarters in Northwood."

His voice turned ragged. "Back at Gordonstoun, he said he would settle for nothing less than a place in the Admiralty. He won't get that by turning down a promotion."

"You were friends once," she reminded him.

"Not after Jonas discovered my father was with the IRA."

She rested her tapered fingers on his sleeve. "You were on opposite sides, but Jonas would never forget a friendship."

"Yet as an officer in the Royal Navy, he would turn me in if he found me here."

"Or be considered a traitor himself," she said softly.

"I never understood why Jonas had such a prominent spot in your life."

"The son of the lord of the manor always has a prominent place. And when his—his mother died, I gave him special care."

"So who is this hanging where my picture used to be?"

"That's Sydney. She was six when that picture was taken. An American businessman and his wife adopted her."

"Lucky girl. Someone wanted her. What about my children?"

"They can spend the night, but in the morning I'll talk to my solicitor about finding a permanent home for them."

"Don't, Abigail. I want them here with you. I trust you."

"I'm doing what's best for Keeley and Danny. I've promised myself for weeks that I would see Edmund Gallagher and make arrangements for the other children and Sir James." She gave him an ironic grin. "Now it's six children instead of four. Your coming now simply brought the need into sharp focus."

I have other legal accounts to settle, she thought. *Funds for Boris's and Griselda's old age. And I must undo what Lady Willoughby did so many years ago—I will sign the property back into Jonas's name.*

"Conon, I won't be here long enough for your children to grow up. One should not live beyond eighty, not when one's strength is failing." She tapped her chest. "Not when I could so easily become a burden for someone else."

She moved along the row of faces. "That's Santos Garibaldi. You remember him? I'm certain you were here at the same time. His father designed the fountain for us." Her voice brightened. "And over here—Sheldon Taylor and Doyle Sullivan. I fretted over those two, but they're both married now and successful."

"They're gone. Don't waste your worries on any of them."

"Sometimes when they're in trouble, they come back. You came back, Conon. Funny, I foolishly thought that one of these boys and his wife could take up my work." She looked over the familiar faces. "But I can't expect someone else to take up my dream. Jonas tells me a dream is distinctly your own. It would no longer be mine if it slipped from my hands."

He didn't move even when Griselda came into the room with a tray of hot dumplings. "Will you hang up my children's pictures?"

"Danny and Keeley won't be here long enough for that," Abigail answered.

"Of course, they will," Griselda said as she turned to leave them. "Two precious children like that. Trust me, Conon O'Reilly, I'll make certain Abigail hangs their pictures with the others. And I won't let Jonas take them down. Now, come and eat your supper while the dumplings are steamy hot."

He gulped down the chicken and dumplings, then wiped his mouth with the back of his hand. Abigail touched his arm. "I wish things could have been different for you. For all of us. But Jonas trusts me. I can't betray him. Jonas checks in on his father before midnight. James grows restless around then."

"Then I'd better leave now. You've taken enough risks for me." As they left the room, he said, "Abigail, are you all right? You look—you look not well again."

"Just another passing flutter," she assured him.

She felt the jerking of her heart. The missed beats. She linked her arm with his and leaned against him.

"Who takes care of the Admiral during the week?" he asked.

"Lucas during the daytime. The Admiral would never think of sending his steward back to Dublin. They get on splendidly. And I stay with the Admiral on the evenings when Jonas isn't here."

"I never understood your great affection for the old man. I thought the British Navy took care of its own."

"They do—but for now, I want him here with me. You used to walk along the river with the Admiral, didn't you?"

Conon's mouth twitched. "A few times."

The evening wind blew cold as she opened the door for him. "Where will you go, Conon?"

He pressed his bristled cheek against hers. "It is best that you don't know, Miss Abigail."

The familiar term of his boyhood. She choked, "I promise you, I won't fail your children. . . . Just stay safe."

"Don't worry. I am invincible."

A patch of moonlight shone faintly in the sky as Conon slipped out the front door. It made him even more of a blackened shadow as he darted into the thickly wooded darkness.

Twigs crackled beneath his booted feet as he edged the well-traversed footpath. She feared lest he stumble and lose his way, but he was already one of her lost ones as he forged his way toward the bridge.

A prayer for Conon stuck in her throat and remained there unuttered. For a frantic moment, she thought to ring Reverend Rainford-Simms and ask him to dash out into the night, over the pedestrian bridge, in search of her lost boy. Wasn't that the clergyman's job—to go after the lost, to rein in the wandering?

A rolling cloud drifted across the moon's path, but Conon would welcome the darkness. The night was too still, filled only with the wingbeats of owls lighting in the conifers, the churning of the waterwheel down by the old mill, and that rippling murmur of the Windrush winding through the rushes. Like the tawny owl, Conon was a creature of the night, given to darkness, his senses alert. But the owl in the woodlands was clothed in thick down; Conon had only his threadworn jacket to warm him.

The sound of his boots on the gravel faded and was gone. She was certain he had reached the fork in the path by now. To his right, he would see a dim light flicker in the chancel of St. Michael's. Charles always left a light on for those in need. But Conon would turn left, away from the redemptive footpath, and make his way stealthily over the old stone bridge to escape from the village of his boyhood.

Without warning, gunfire shattered the stillness.

She stumbled down the steps. "Conon, Conon."

A sharp pain like a knuckled fist furrowed across her chest. She gripped the rail to regain her footing. As the sharpness eased, she cried again, "Conon, Conon!"

Only the rustling wind and gurgling river answered her. With her heart still knocking unevenly, she forced herself back up the steps—determined to protect Danny and Keeley. She put her trembling hand on the brass knob and shoved the door open. More gunfire split the spring air. She saw

Griselda running down the hall toward her, heard Gregor's cry as he ran beside Griselda.

Another explosion erupted behind Abigail. Closer this time. A crushing pain seared through her back and chest. For a second she stood motionless, stunned. Griselda's face blurred.

The tingling began in her fingers. Numbness. Utter help-lessness as pain radiated into her jaw. The weight on her chest grew heavier. Unbearable. She tried to grasp Griselda's hand, to smile at Gregor. Then all awareness slipped from her as she slumped to the cold, dank floor of the manor.

Five

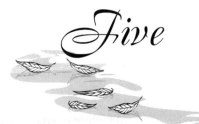

In Washington, time lagged eight hours behind the Cotswold clocks. Sydney awakened at dawn on Saturday with a metallic jangle blaring in her ears, her unlisted number ringing off the hook. It had to be Randolph calling at this unearthly hour to apologize—or to make excuses—for their latest lovers' quarrel.

She could hear him now, nonchalantly suggesting that he join her at the Barrington retreat in the woods for the weekend. Deliberately pretending the quarrel didn't matter. Thanks to her parents he had always had a room of his own, had always been welcomed as part of the family. He still had a key and thought nothing of popping in at unexpected moments, more so since their engagement. At those times, when the loss of her parents seemed the most poignant, Randolph was comforting to have around. Sadly though, Randy would remain the man her parents had trusted, the one they wanted for a son-in-law. Their choice. Not hers.

Dear Randy. Tall, trim, his eyes a cold gray-blue last evening. He was so much like her father. Shrewd in business, he'd earned his first million before he was thirty and now, at thirty-eight, thanks to her father's investment tips, was working on his second million. A well-groomed man, but no matter what his attire, he wore his emotions up front. Ardor. Impatience. Disappointment.

The phone rang for the third time. She ignored it, concentrating on the extravagance that surrounded her—a king-size bed, a Jacuzzi tub, and a spacious, pink dressing room only steps away. She owned her own home, held the top post at Barrington Enterprises, and traveled abroad frequently. What more could Randolph Iverson offer her?

Mother Nature flooded her room with brilliance as the sun broke through the wispy clouds. But Sydney kept rehashing the quarrel. Randolph wanted a commitment from her. She gazed somberly at his photo on her bedside table. He was an intriguing mixture—Jew and Gentile, two worlds wrapped into one man. His piercing eyes and spirited way of speaking came from his mother; the narrow, irregular nose and angular face from his dad.

In an unguarded moment, shortly after her parents' accident, Sydney had accepted Randolph Iverson's ring. But in truth, she didn't want to get married. She had everything she needed or could possibly want. Books and music and art were matters that she could share with Randolph. But not their hearts, their lives. Not her love of the woods and the river. And not that secret yearning that lingered at the edge of consciousness, tantalizing her with longings for something special, impressions that she could not identify.

On rare occasions, when she ventured to share her heart and dreams with him, he'd tug his ear and laugh uproariously. "You and your Shangri-La. Your Garden of Eden. It doesn't exist, sweetheart." But she knew he was wrong.

Love him? Sometimes she loathed him. Last night's blowup had come over her mother's sewing room. She rehearsed their bitter words, Randolph's thin lips pursed, his voice soothing, languid.

"Sydney, it's time to think about us. Get the house cleared out so it can be our house. Finish going through your mother's things and put her to rest."

"That's not fair. I can't risk the memories it will stir."

"And you're not being fair to us. You can't bring your mother back."

By mid-morning, Sydney took the key and unlocked the door to her mother's sewing room. As she stepped inside, she was struck with an overwhelming sense of her mother's presence. The silent room echoed with the remembered sounds of her mother's humming and the clacking treadle of the sewing machine. The brightly lit room still held the faint scent of her mother's fragrant sachets.

The shelves across the room were filled with dolls that Millicent Barrington had prepared for the children at the local hospital. The apple-cheeked china doll in a fleecy robe. The rag doll in denim overalls. And the old-fashioned porcelain one dressed in taffeta and lace—the doll that Sydney had promised to give away to someone special.

Sydney swept the room with a singular gaze. Everything was exactly as her mother had left it. The Swiss-made sewing machine faced the bay windows. Spools of thread hung from wooden spindles, their bright colors ribboned like a rainbow on the wall. A bolt of gingham leaned against one corner, and doll patterns lay strewn on the worktable. The polished armoire stood open, revealing more drawers and shelves crammed with buttons, zippers, and scraps of flannel and broadcloth. Even the rug by the sewing machine bore the imprint of Sydney's hours of sitting there watching her mother's fingers move deftly, lovingly as she formed intricate doll garments.

Her mother's pink slippers lay sprawled by the foot pedal—lying in the spot where she had kicked them off the night before her flight to Europe. Sydney caught her own reflection in the mirror on the armoire. How lost she looked. A lump rose in her throat as she crossed the room to the sewing machine where a square of velour was held securely under the pressure foot—the beginnings of a doll dress that her mother never finished.

Slipping into her mother's chair, Sydney looked out on the yard and beyond toward the Olympic Mountains. Her mother had been a private person—deep, caring, sensitive.

Her father she understood better—a proud, public figure concerned about his image. She was so much like him—skillful at wielding a strong arm at Barrington Enterprises, emanating his power and strength.

But she had so little of her mother's gentleness. She ran her fingers over the sewing machine, removing a layer of dust from it. Her mother had been content to stay in the background, yet at the sound of her husband's BMW roaring into the driveway or his footsteps on the gravel, Millicent always stopped what she was doing and hurried to meet him.

The room, so much a part of her mother, brought back the last moments they had spent here together. Millicent's soft words seemed to fill the room. "Is Randolph coming to dinner this evening?" she had asked.

"Probably. He never waits for an invitation. This morning Daddy asked me when I was going to marry him so he could just move in permanently. Imagine!"

"Your father doesn't believe in long engagements." She laughed happily. "Ours, as you know, was quite short-lived."

"Randolph and I are not engaged."

"I'm certain he's asked you. So what's it going to take?"

"A bombshell."

Her mother concentrated on stitching the tiny doll dress. "What did you tell your father, Sydney?"

"That I cherish my independence, the freedom to come and go as I please. I just can't tie up my life to one person."

Millicent paused in her sewing. "Is that how you view your father and me? Tied up? Without freedom?"

Her parents—so different, so in love. Aaron, the dashing, keen-witted businessman, silver-haired as far back as Sydney could remember. And Millicent, the beautiful and graceful wife with the soft English accent at his side. "You're different, Mom. You don't object to doing things Dad's way. You think alike. No matter what Daddy wants, you go along with it."

Slowly, Millicent turned to face her daughter, her eyes sad. "You have it all wrong, dear. Aaron and I do things together because we love each other. I like pleasing him, and at the end of a harried day at the office, he finds comfort in coming home to me. He still courts me with roses. A world without your father in it would be dreadfully lonely."

"It's not like that with Randy and me. Randolph doesn't have Dad's charisma. I just can't explain him—"

"Can you explain yourself?" her mother had asked. "Do you know your own heart, know what you want?"

"Sometimes."

But how could she explain to Millicent that sometimes she found Randy charming, attentive, a comforting companion? Yet, if he left town in the morning, her world would still go on. It would never be that way with her parents. They needed each other.

"I was sixteen when Dad first brought Randy home to dinner. I guess I just think of him as a friend."

Her mother paused in her stitching and smiled. "I saw right away that he was your father's kind of man. Intelligent. A quick learner. We liked him. Your father would like him as a son-in-law." She matched a spool of thread against the material in her hand. "But I want you to be happy, so choose carefully, Sydney."

It's coming now, she thought. The mother-daughter lecture that Sydney had outgrown long ago. *Preserve yourself for the one you love.* But what if you never fell in love?

Her mother's foot balanced above the treadle, caught in space, caught in time. She glanced down at Sydney. "If you don't plan to marry—don't plan to give Aaron and me grandchildren—what is it you want to do with your life, dear?"

Sydney drew her knees to her chest. "Dad insists that I take over Barrington Enterprises if anything happens to him. Randolph won't like that. He thinks Dad promised the job to him."

"Aaron wants a Barrington in charge. You'll be good at it, my bright little feather. With your master's in aerospace engineering, you're a genius with figures and you understand business mergers and government contracts. You've always been your daddy's girl. He's trained you well."

She switched to a blue thread. "But promise me you won't let the position and power at Barrington destroy you."

"Destroy me? Mother, I plan to grow rich working there."

"We have already made you rich. Someday, you will own this house as well. When you're talking with Aaron about defense plants and government contracts, you're efficient. Even ruthless at times. But when you're with me at the hospital, passing out the dolls to the children, you remind me of Dulcie. You'd make a fine pediatric doctor or nurse—like Dulcie was before she went to Africa."

She cupped Sydney's cheek. "More and more, you look like your mother. Dulcie was beautiful and so are you. You have her facial features and a bit of her gentleness. And you have your father's strong points too. He was very intelligent—as you are."

"Why do you never talk about my birth parents?"

"I am now. Aaron doesn't like being reminded that you were not our flesh and blood."

"But I am yours. You and Dulcie were sisters. And Dad shouldn't feel bad. A lot of people say I look like Aaron. I love him; he's the only father I've ever known."

Millicent held up a finished dress of taffeta and lace for inspection. Putting it on the empress doll, she said, "Won't this make some child happy?"

"It's adorable, Mother. Randolph teased me last night about having a mother who still played with dolls so late in life."

"You tell Randolph Iverson that I never had a doll of my own in those years after the war. Never." Her eyes grew misty. "Syd, dear, I want you to give this one away to someone special."

"We'll do that on our next visit to the children's ward."

"I won't have time to deliver it before my trip to Europe."

"It can keep till you get back."

"No, promise me." She reflected. "When your father and I get back from this business trip abroad, let's the two of us plan a vacation. I'll take you back to England to the place where Dulcie and I were born. And to the church where she was married."

"I'd like that. Would Dad mind?"

"Very much so. But this is something I should have done a long time ago. You need to know more about your birth parents. We've given you everything, and yet I feel we have let you down. I don't know what you really want to do with your life. No, that's not true. You have always talked of working with children—of leaving your position at Barrington. But I guess I just went along with Aaron's dreams for you."

Her brows puckered. "If you left Barrington, what would you want to do? Tell me and I'll try and talk to Aaron while we're in Europe. It will be hard to make him understand—he has his heart so set on you working beside him, but he loves you—"

Sydney knew that she was groping for something abstract, something undefined. Something she couldn't explain to her parents because it had no label. But surely it would include children. "I haven't worked out anything definite. But I think I'll recognize the right place when I find it."

"Are you thinking about God, Sydney?"

"What does God have to do with my future?"

Her mother's eyes watered. "Everything, perhaps. I really have failed you. Failed myself. Aaron has never been a very religious man—so I never pushed that part of your training."

"I've turned out all right." But even as she said it, she sensed an aching void inside.

"I should stay home this time, but Aaron likes me to travel with him. I'm glad you're flying as far as New York with us though."

"Can't miss a chance for a shopping spree. And I want to be at Kennedy International to make sure you get on that plane."

Sydney remembered that wistful look on her mother's face when she hugged her good-bye at the Kennedy boarding gate.

"Sydney, darling, you'll be all right by yourself?"

"Of course. Don't be ridiculous. I'm a grown woman."

But she had wept like a little child moments later as news spread through the airport terminal that her parents' jet had just crashed in Long Island Sound, minutes after takeoff.

Sydney shook off those memories and concentrated on a large black spider crawling across the floor in the sewing room. In search, she was certain, of a refuge of its own. With clarity, she knew her mother was right. She was searching for her own person, her own self. How could she discover who she really was if she married Randolph? They could never be one. Never.

Hours later Sydney sat curled on the floor in her white shorts and a T-shirt, her face and hands dirt-smudged, her nostrils filled with layers of dust. The fuzz from a tangle of spiderwebs curled on her bare leg as she sorted through her mother's things. A growing pile of toss-aways lay to her left: old patterns, mismatched buttons, scraps of fabric that Millicent Barrington could have turned into doll clothing. On her right, Sydney had stacked craft books and the awards her mother had won for dolls she had made.

Tearing the last carton open, she waded through a layer of yellowed newsprint before finding an old album—the pictorial record of her mother's childhood in post-war London, her mother's adult life before Aaron. In one unlabeled snapshot, her mother and three friends stood arm-in-arm in front of Lake Geneva. In another, they ran hand-in-hand over crusted snow in Austria. These were friends that her mother had lost touch with after her marriage. Aaron Quinton Barrington had not only swept into Millicent's life at a London ball, he had whisked her out of London and away from everything English, everything familiar.

Sydney studied the last picture in the album—a picture of herself as a small child standing in front of the Barringtons in the middle of an English garden. Aaron was looking into the camera—smiling, dark-haired, handsome. Her mother wore a wide-brimmed hat, her dark-lashed eyes peering out beneath the rim. On a sloping hill in the distance stood a large country house with a river winding below it. Sydney could not recall being there, but she remembered the gurgling, bubbling sound of the river.

Six

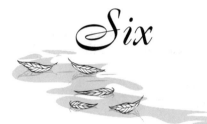

In his cottage on the Broadshire property, Jonas Willoughby crouched in front of the stone fireplace, set a match to the kindling, and watched the fire flame and crackle. Satisfied with the roaring fire, he stood and was confronted at once with Louise's photograph on the mantel.

Her lips were parted, smiling. Smiling at him when he snapped that picture. He traced the lines of her face, missing her as he did. He opened his mouth to call her name—to have her come and share the fire with him, and at once remembered that no matter how much he called, she would never come to him again.

Here in the Cotswolds, in the most peaceful place he had ever known, he couldn't shake off the uncertainty of interfering in other lives, of having them interfere in his own. He felt tormented at the thought of placing his father in a permanent residence. Undecided about Abigail and Gregor. Annoyed by Griselda's silent disapproval. His own bitterness with the IRA had almost destroyed his communion with himself and his God. And Charles—that man of peace—remained a constant reminder of what might have been. Thoughts of all of them crowded his daytime hours out on the wolds. Thundered in his ears when he played his bagpipes. Invaded his dreams at night, turning them into nightmares.

Jonas kicked off his boots and sagged into his recliner. At midnight he would cross the grounds to the manor and sit by his father's bedside until dawn. For now, it was good to stretch and close his eyes and sleep—a sleep deep and troubled as it propelled him back into the days before Louise, to the days without her. Back to the job he loved more than anything—into a sweeping panorama of the past, of flying, of launching his Sea Harrier off the flight deck of the *HMS Invincible*.

It was the same dream.

The same nightmare.

In the moonlight, the deck of the aircraft carrier gleamed like silver. The ordnance handlers had loaded the Amraam missiles. The deck crew signaled for takeoff. Jonas gave a gloved thumbs-up and with his Pegasus jet engine running full throttle, the Harrier screamed into the vast emptiness of the sky, leaving the carrier swallowed in darkness.

Squinting owlishly through the canopy toward the wingtip, Jonas saw only empty space. The hazy swirling clouds left the sky a cinereous gray. Jonas was flying blind on a combat patrol to Yugoslavia. Flying alone, his squadron nowhere in sight. He tried to rally the control tower. Silence. He felt confused, his oxygen depleted. He was totally alone.

It was impossible to turn the plane back.

The menacing silhouette of the Harrier roared on toward Kosovo, rapidly closing the gap as its onboard computers scanned for a target. Gregor's village lay ahead and he must blow it into cinders, root out the Serbs who had dug in there. He had his mission, his Amraam missiles. As Jonas activated the weapons system, the cockpit screen showed "target acquired," then "locked." His thumb hovered over the firing button, just waiting for the moment.

He tried to identify the target, but the weather had turned murky. Gregor's village? He couldn't fire on Gregor's village. In the semidarkness outside his canopy, he spotted the Serb interceptor zeroing in on him—a Russian-built MiG–29 fighter, the pilot faceless. Just then, the Serb climbed erratically. From the ground came the burst of antiaircraft guns and surface-to-air missiles. The explosions erupted around the Harrier in orange and white flames. Jonas fixed his gaze on the panel in front of him and fought for control. Pushing buttons. Twirling knobs. He was like a white knuckler, an anxious passenger in the pilot's seat.

The MiG–29 screamed toward him again, the face in the cockpit taking form now. Young like himself. A man without a face mask. For a moment Jonas knew dread, the fear of dying. Heart pounding fear. He pressed his thumb onto the firing button. Heard the explosion. Saw more flames engulfing him. He was forced to maintain radio silence with no one but God on his wingtip.

"Abort. Abort!" he told himself.

The ejection seat jammed. He was locked in, spiraling downward. He would welcome death if he could see Louise again. No, he wanted to go on living. His skill was being tested to the limit; his survivorship training kicked in. Hope rose. He knew deep in the ship, in the operations room, seamen were monitoring his Harrier, tracking him on the radar screen—the rotating blades of radar swinging back and forth.

His arms ached as he tried to level the plane. He needed some assurance that God was flying this one out with him. "Our Father who art in heaven. . . ."

Was that how it went? Is that how you prayed when you were nose diving into eternity? No, something more direct. Zero straight in. Abigail maintained that God always listened.

"God," he mouthed beneath his mask. "Let me live. Take me safely back to the carrier. No, take me back to Gregor so I can tell him that someone else destroyed his village."

Spiraling through a patch of drifting clouds, he was convinced that he was over the Emerald Island, close to the narrow road where Louise had been ambushed. He saw motion beneath him. The IRA stronghold. Not Serbs, but the IRA terrorists. His muddled brain refused to clear. With a quick maneuver, he leveled out, gained altitude. At 600 knots he seemed to creak along. Going nowhere. Unable to turn the plane back to the Adriatic Sea.

Jonas felt a rush of cold over his legs and had time to wonder why he wasn't wearing his flying boots. He reached for the zipper on his flying suit and felt instead the soft twill of his tweed jacket. As he breathed deeply into his oxygen mask, the smell of country and sheep and wild thyme filled his nostrils. Suddenly his seat shot forward, his legs extended. He tried to right himself and felt his dog nuzzling the back of his hand.

Jonas came out of his nightmare sweating, his lanky body pressed against the back of the recliner. He was in his thatched cottage on the edge of the Broadshire property. Safe. Alive. He had been dreaming.

He blinked against the grogginess, his mind still reeling from the nightmare: Kosovo; the ship; taking off in his Harrier jet. But that was a year or two ago, part of the past. His duty. His duty to kill innocent people. He massaged his throbbing temples. When he flew the sorties, the Kosovo bombings had exploded in his ears. They still resounded in his thoughts. He glanced at his watch, surprised that he had slept only five minutes. Ten at most. A mere fragment of time in his thirty-four years. Yet he had just spent a season in hell, a torturous journey into war.

What had sent him into this mental tailspin? Thoughts of Louise? No, thoughts of Gregor walking beside him today out on the knoll, saying, "Lucas said you bombed my papa's village. Will my papa ever come home again?"

Gamely, Jonas had tried to explain to the boy about war. Tried to tell man-to-boy why the Allied Forces had flown sorties over his country. Why did it matter now? Gregor had been little more than seven then, an evacuee trucked across the border into Macedonia. No, that wasn't what happened. Gregor had been forced to walk the last ten miles toward the border with one shoe gone. Somewhere between his own troubled country and the refugee camp near Skopje, the Albanian guerrilla thrust the frightened child, without kin or a tin of water, into Abigail's waiting arms.

Wood cracked in the stone fireplace and slipped in charred blackness through the iron grate. TopGun's wet nose nudged his hand again, then the dog raced to the cottage door whimpering.

Outside, an explosion shattered the stillness of early evening. Jonas's bare feet hit the floor before he realized he was standing. The explosion had been real, the dream unreal. Something out of the ordinary was happening down by the Windrush. He wiggled into his boots, stumbled out of the cottage, and ran toward the river with his collie at his heels.

Now the sound of angry voices gave him new direction. When he came within yards of the bridge, he was convinced that the entire village had turned out. Women and children stood in the background, too curious to go back to the safety of their cottages. Men huddled in groups, staring at the ground. The gurgle of the river went steadily on, flowing down the center of town and winding peacefully over the valley.

"Jonas."

Even in the darkness, he recognized the gangly man beside him. At six-feet-two, Jonas rarely felt stunted in another man's presence, but Charles Rainford-Simms, in spite of his stooped shoulders, had two inches on him. Charles was in shirt sleeves with an unbuttoned vest, his clerical collar loose at his neck.

"Charles, I heard gunfire. What happened here?"

"A young man—a stranger in town—was shot. But he escaped."

"We rarely have strangers in town, Charles. Who was he?"

"I thought you would know."

Jonas scanned the crowd milling around in tight-knit groups. The pub owner waved his flashlight toward the thicket. "Here. Over here!" he cried. His beam of light centered on a patch of ground by the river. He lifted his hand. "Blood," he said. "We've got him. He can't be far—he's losing too much blood."

The schoolmaster took up the cry. "You women, go home. Take the children with you and lock the doors."

Lock the doors? Jonas shrugged. *How many people in the village even have locks on their doors?*

The schoolmaster thundered more orders. "Nigel, take some men with you and scour the thicket. Peter, take a group and fan out on the other side of the river. Two or three of you stay with me. We'll follow the Windrush on this side." He glanced at Charles. "No need for you to come. We younger men can take care of everything. Go back to the church in case you are needed."

Jonas started forward to join the schoolmaster. Charles pulled him back. "You heard him. The villagers can handle it." He kept a restraining hand on Jonas's arm. "Let the others go. Neither one of us should be there, not if there's more gunfire. Besides, son, I must talk to you."

Jonas spun on his heels. "We can talk later."

"No, you see, the wounded man is not the only stranger in town. Two gentlemen called on me earlier this afternoon."

Jonas rubbed the collie's head. "Visiting bishops?"

"Hardly. Intelligence officers. MI5, would be my guess."

For the first time since coming home, Jonas felt uneasy. Had three years of grieving robbed Charles of his quick wit? Or was Mrs. Quigley right? "He seems a bit dotty at times, muttering and puttering in his garden," she had said.

"Intelligence officers, Charles? That's highly unlikely in Stow-on-the-Woodland. Unless—"

"Unless they were looking for you or me." Charles watched him with wise old eyes. "My boy, I know the rumors, but I have my wits about me. So don't tell me to retire and take that long-deserved rest. That long rest will come soon enough."

Doggedly, Jonas persisted. "How old are you now?"

"On my birthday three years ago I turned seventy-five; I haven't counted since then, but I'm not too old to know that those men were snooping around our village when I invited them in for tea."

"Charles, later. Please. I must join the others."

"You must not get involved. You see, when I showed the visitors my model train, they admitted that they were looking for an Irish agent living in this village. I refused to allow them to use the sanctity of the church to search for anyone. And they knew that I was Louise's father—said they expected more cooperation from me since my daughter died at the hands of Irish terrorists."

He touched the collar around his neck, pure white even in the darkness. "I am committed to helping people, not destroying them. But if they're right—if there is an Irish terrorist in the village—if this has anything to do with Louise, then those strangers may be looking for you. You must leave at once, Jonas, and go back to Northwood. Go back tonight."

Jonas jammed his hands deep into his pockets. "I'm not a man who runs. I know you believe what you're saying, but whatever is happening here this evening has nothing to do with me or Louise."

Charles rocked thoughtfully on his heels. "I was wrong to keep you from joining the search party. I'm sorry. But I've been missing you. Surely you remember your way to the vicarage? You must." His voice cracked. "Someone has been putting flowers on Louise's grave. You, perhaps? Even so, you don't stop by for a visit with me. We used to play chess together. I'd enjoy a game."

"I'll make it a point to come next weekend."

From the shadows, they saw Boris hurrying toward them. "Commander, go to the house. Miss Broderick needs you. Doctor Wallis is on his way."

As Jonas and the dog raced toward the manor, Charles heard the search party shouting in the distance. He turned in the direction of the church, an uneasiness tingling his spine. He was accustomed to long walks alone at night, roaming the Cotswold Hills. Praying. Singing. Worshipping his God. But as he moved toward the vicarage, a voice called sharply from the darkness.

"Reverend. Over here, by the trees."

Rainford-Simms stared without seeing. "Who are you?"

A whispered answer. "Lucas, Admiral Willoughby's steward."

Charles almost stumbled over the body lying on the ground.

"I need your help, Reverend. This man is badly wounded."

Charles knelt down, and with his penlight, studied the troubled young face grimacing in pain. His light trailed to the man's blood-soaked jacket and shirt. "We're here, son." And to Lucas, "He needs a doctor. All I'd have to do is ring the church bell and the men searching for him will come back."

"I daren't allow that. The crowd is merciless. I can treat a gunshot wound, Reverend. Just help me get him to safety. You must help me. . . . He's one of Miss Broderick's boys."

Stunned, Charles asked, "Does she know he's in town?"

"Does it matter? You are a man of the cloth, and this man needs a sanctuary, sir. If we hurry, we can get him to the church before the villagers come back."

The man went limp as they pulled him to his feet. "We won't get far, dragging him like this. He'll only bleed more."

"But, Reverend, we can't let him die in the bushes."

Blood splashed on Charles's clothes. Time was running short. "There's a trout stream that branches off from the Windrush. It flows just beneath the vicarage. Do you know where I mean?"

"That's a tangled mess of bracken and underbrush. We can never get through."

"There is always a way through. The vines hide a footpath from the bank to the vicarage. It's too much for an old man to climb often, but if you help me, we can make it. It is the only way to let the Windrush wash away our bloody footprints." As they struggled up the trail, he asked, "Why do you want to help him? Are we not breaking the laws of the land?"

"I told you, he's one of Abigail Broderick's boys. And, Reverend, I am like you. I no longer bear arms or take sides. I've been the Admiral's steward for far too long."

"But you have political convictions?"

"Aye. That I do." He feigned a Gaelic twang as they stopped to catch their breath. "I've lived all my life in England, but I was born an Irishman, sir. And this man is one of my countrymen."

An icy knot formed in Charles's stomach. *The IRA? A young terrorist?* He was breaking the laws of the village, the rules of the church. Perhaps the laws of his God. Could he skim by on the Good Samaritan clause taking this man into the vicarage?

"God forgive me for getting involved," he said.

"God bless you for getting involved."

As they neared the vicarage, the door swung back, casting a bright light on their path. A young woman in an artist's apron appeared on the landing. "Oh, it's you, Reverend! What is all this thrashing about in the bushes?" she scolded. "Have you gone quite mad trying to find your way home?"

Lucas stiffened. "Who are you?"

She pushed strands of hair from her cheek with a paintbrush. "Kersten. Surely you remember me, Lucas. I do light housekeeping for the reverend in exchange for room and board."

He asked gruffly, "Does your light housekeeping include helping an injured man?"

Kersten pocketed the paintbrush and rubbed her paint-smudged fingers. "So that's what all the shouting is about? Come in quickly so I can darken the windows. Who is he, Reverend?"

"One of Miss Broderick's lost boys."

"Poor man. Can't be all bad if he belongs to Miss Abigail. And, Lucas, I am good at boiling water."

She stood aside to let them enter, shock registering in her expression at the sight of the man's ashen face and bloody jacket. Then quite calmly, she said, "He's bleeding badly—but I'm good at washing up."

"We can trust her," Charles said.

And the door closed on the darkness outside.

"Stay, TopGun," Jonas commanded.

The collie obeyed as Jonas sprinted up the steps of the manor and flung back the door. As he stepped inside, Gregor flew into his arms.

"Has something happened to Sir James, Gregor?"

"No, it's . . . it's Miss Abigail."

He pushed the boy aside and bounded up the curving stairs, his lanky legs taking three steps at a time. He was breathless when he reached Abigail's room. She lay on her bed, her eyes closed, her arms limp at her sides. The periwinkle blue comforter that he had given her at Christmas had been drawn to her waist. Her silver-gray hair—always neatly in place—sprawled loosely on the pillow. Jonas felt like an intruder, invading her privacy.

"Abby."

She moaned, mumbling indistinct words. He felt a surge of relief that she was alive. He strode across the room and took her icy hand in his. Her lips were blue, her skin milk-white. When he called her name again, she gave him a ghost of a smile.

"Abby, what happened?"

"My heart."

He pressed his fingers to her wrist and felt her pulse. "Dr. Wallis is coming."

Tears filled her eyes. He knuckled them away. "Did he make it, Jonas?"

"Who, Abby?"

Griselda was standing on the other side of the bed now. "The gunfire upset her. You must leave at once. Go back to London."

"I can't run out on Abigail."

Abigail's eyelids fluttered open again. "Please go."

Griselda chewed her lower lip. "There's nothing you can do here. Abigail doesn't want you involved—"

"Involved in what?"

"Just go. I will call you." He heard the sob in Griselda's voice. Saw the proud chin jut forward. "It's what Abigail wants. She wants you safe, Jonas."

"I can't leave her—not like this."

"And you can't do anything for her, except pray. You can do that on the way back to Northwood."

Pray? Abigail's beliefs no longer rubbed off on him. He stared down at the woman who had prayed for him all of his life—the woman who had been at the family manor whenever he went home from Gordonstoun or Dartmouth or on leave from the Navy. He choked up at the thought of her dying. She had watched him grow to manhood, had an unflinching pride in him and always words of wisdom or rebuke when he went home. She was right, of course. A man couldn't travel the rough seas or fly into battle without knowing that someone bigger than himself had charted the universe and tempered the seas. It wasn't Abigail's fault he had shelved God.

"If the Admiral were well, he'd order you to go," Griselda remarked.

Jonas leaned down and kissed Abigail on the forehead. "I'll be back next weekend—or the one after that. Get well, Abby."

Exhausted, she whispered, "Take the back roads."

He glanced at Griselda. "What is she saying?"

"She wants you to go the back roads, then join up with A-40 and on into London. With the ruckus that's going on, the police will stop anyone going through the main towns—and discover that you are from Northwood and NATO Intelligence."

Gently, he laid Abigail's hand against the comforter. When he reached the door, he heard Boris and Doctor Wallis coming up the stairs. Jonas crossed the hall and ducked into an empty room. Once they had stepped into Abigail's bedroom, Jonas went quietly down the back steps to his cottage.

Gregor was sitting in Jonas's recliner, his arms around the dog. "You're going away?" he accused.

"For a few days." Jonas threw his things into the kit bag. "Will you take care of TopGun for me while I'm gone?"

The boy nodded. "Will Miss Abigail die, Jonas?"

Jonas bent to spread the ashes in the fireplace. Picking up the daily paper, he tossed it in his case. Then, as he turned out the lights, he said, "I don't know, Gregor."

"I'm scared, Jonas."

"We both are." He put his arm around the boy and led him out the cottage door. "Go back to the house and get some sleep, son. Take TopGun with you."

"Mrs. Quigley won't let TopGun into the house."

"She will tonight. She'll understand."

He tossed his luggage in the car. "Gregor, Miss Abigail doesn't want anyone to know I was here this weekend."

Gregor sniffed and wiped his nose with the back of his hand. "I know. Mrs. Quigley told me."

$\mathcal{S}$even

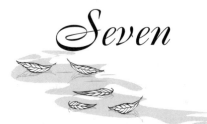

Sydney stepped out onto the lower deck of the rustic retreat where she had come to spend the weekend. Everything she owned bore the signature of Aaron Barrington and spoke of wealth. The four-bedroom house with its knotty-pine siding and wide, wraparound porch sat high on a bluff overlooking the river. She ran her fingers over the beveled porch railing and thought of her father standing there, loving nature, loving life.

He had stood in that very spot when she, as a sixteen-year-old, had rushed outside, exclaiming, "Dad, now that school is out, I'm going to train for the marathon."

His grip on the railing tightened. "A race? Honey, the Barringtons don't waste a whole summer running. You're going to be managing the company someday."

"But it's a benefit for children with AIDS. I talked to Mother about it. I've signed up; I've given my word."

"Your mother didn't discuss it with me. She knows I'm holding a place at Barrington Enterprises for you this summer."

"Dad, don't your employees have to be eighteen?"

"You won't be on the payroll. With your genius for math, I've arranged a special apprenticeship for you in the engineering department. You'll learn the business firsthand—"

"I'm not needed there. I'm needed in the marathon. Don't you understand? It would mean something if Aaron Barrington's daughter won the race."

He reached into his back pocket and whipped out his checkbook. "I'll make a contribution. What about five thousand? Who do I make it out to?"

She fought back hot tears. "Is it worth that much to buy my place in the race?"

"It is to me, Sydney."

Yes, worth it, she thought, *to always have your own way.*

Sydney wondered why such searing memories of her father attacked so often. She dragged one of the patio chairs over with her bare foot and sank down in its padded comfort. Her father bought everything with money, but he couldn't buy time. Now that she had his money at her disposal, she wanted only those things that wealth could not buy: solitude, peace, contentment.

From the cabin to the river, nature was garbed in spring colors. Flimsy tree branches turning a buttercup yellow. Bushes and hedges in a patchwork of holly and Kendal green on the upper cliffs. The weeping willows in shades of moss and lime, bending gracefully toward the water's edge.

Sydney had spent her whole life on the river. A privileged kid—swimming, boating, water-skiing, riding her horse along the mountain streams. Listening to the gurgling sound of the river, she felt as though life had turned normal again. But it hadn't. She rubbed her finger where the diamond had been a week ago.

Why had she accepted Randolph's proposal so soon after her parents' death? Out of loneliness? Because he was her father's choice? Randolph was always there to field her questions, to laugh and talk with, to dine with on quiet evenings. As her fiancé, he went on being a welcomed guest at the Barrington home and at the cabin, their long friendship as cozy and comfortable as a warm fire. But it had been a fiery good-bye.

"You're married to the job, Syd. I can't compete against that."

"Then don't," she had snapped. "The job is only a temporary arrangement until something better comes along. Someone better."

His jaw had tightened as he stared at the diamond in his hand. "Sydney, would you recognize love if the right person walked into your life?"

She didn't know.

In her mind, she saw him running down the front steps of her home on Lake Washington. She could still hear the door of his Jaguar slam. His tires squeal. She knew he loved her. But no matter how she tried, she did not love him. Why then did the thought of walking back into the empty cabin right now fill her with dread? Tonight, with so many friends a phone call away, she would be alone, with only the sounds of the river and nature to comfort her. She admitted to herself the inner longing to really belong to someone special, to love as her parents had loved. But she knew no one who could fill the void of an empty house, an empty heart.

In the midst of her dark musings, the phone rang. It had to be Randolph. On the eighth ring she picked up the receiver.

"Hello. Sydney speaking," she said guardedly.

"Mrs. Barrington?" The accent sounded decidedly British.

"*Miss* Barrington," she corrected.

"This is Edmund Gallagher from the Gallagher, Blackstone, and Rentley firm in London, England."

A lawyer? A problem at one of their overseas facilities?

Solemnly, he said, "I was Abigail Broderick's solicitor."

She wanted to say, *And who is that?*

"Miss Barrington, our connection is a bit garbled."

She switched the receiver to her other hand and amused herself by counting her polished toes. "I'm still here."

With dignity, he said, "It is my sad duty to inform you that Miss Broderick is dead."

"Dead?" she repeated.

"Yes, I am so sorry."

No need to be sorry, she thought. *I don't know any Abigail Broderick.* At least she did not remember the name. Did not know whether she was a distant relative on her mother's side or one of her mother's old friends.

"What happened to her, Mr. Gallagher?"

"A heart attack. Miss Broderick died in her own manor."

In her own manner. Who would choose a heart attack? Did that run in the family? On the Barrington side? Her mother's side? No. Dulcie, her mother's only known relative, was dead.

"It was quick," the solicitor said.

The garbled distraction on the wire pierced her ear as though Gallagher had run a silver coin across the mouth-piece. The words of the man on the other end of the line sounded distorted.

"Miss Broderick had been unwell for some time, and as far as we can determine, Miss Barrington, Abigail Broderick has left everything to you."

Stunned, Sydney tried to absorb the fact that she had just inherited some stranger's possessions when she was already rich and needed nothing. In her mind, she conjured up an elegant old house on the Thames or a Tudor manor. Then curiosity took over. Why had the Barringtons not told her about this woman?

"Perhaps you can be a little more explicit, Mr. Gallagher?"

"Regarding the inheritance? It includes a house and a walled property with an English garden. Stables—"

A house and a garden. Again Sydney envisioned a lovely home on the River Thames. Or a Chelsea residence off King's Road—a place to stay on her trips abroad. But stables in London? Ashamed of her mental wanderings, her thoughts turned back to the unknown woman with a heart too weak to keep on beating.

"Was Miss Broderick elderly?" she asked.

She heard the rattle of papers. "Quite so. Late seventies."

"Is her property in London? You said you were calling from there."

"No, the property is in the Cotswolds. It's called the Broadshire Manor. Quite a substantial place in the village of Stow-on-the-Woodland. You have heard of it?"

"No, not really. . . . And the truth is, Mr. Gallagher, I don't know anyone named Broderick. I don't even know for certain whether we have relatives in England. And certainly no stranger would leave her things to me."

He raised his voice. "I am a careful man, Miss Barrington. It seems unlikely that I have the wrong number or have dialed the wrong person."

So! She was talking to a man who didn't make mistakes. He seemed so indifferent, so uncaring as he spoke of his client. Sydney pictured Edmund Gallagher sitting self-righteously at his desk, drumming his fingers on Abigail Broderick's will. As his words droned on, she wondered how well he knew Miss Broderick. Or was he simply discharging his duty as her lawyer? She imagined him well-attired in a suit tailored on Chancery Lane and decided that he no doubt took his law degree on the West End and had his plush office tucked in somewhere among England's white-wigged barristers.

Gallagher cleared his throat. For a moment there was no static on the line. "I have Miss Broderick's file in front of me. You are the daughter of Aaron and Millicent Barrington. Correct? Your father was a business icon? Known worldwide? Made his money in the defense program. Correct?"

He rattled off her birth date, her age, her educational attainments, including her summer at Oxford and those marvelous nine months studying French in Paris. Then quite cagily he said, "Perhaps you met Miss Broderick while you studied at Oxford? Or, I see from a notation here that your tie-in with Miss Broderick might go back to a missionary couple in Africa."

It was more than she wanted him to know about her. "Go on."

"Are you certain your parents never mentioned Miss Broderick?"

"If they did, I've forgotten."

The suspicion in the back of her mind intensified. She twisted the telephone cord, longing for the opportunity to ask the operator to trace the call. Gallagher could be a crackpot, someone aware of the value of Barrington Enterprises. Someone aware that she was at the cabin alone with a chilling breeze blowing up from the river. She curled her legs under her to warm her feet, but the sudden chill remained.

"I am upsetting you with news of Miss Broderick's death," the solicitor said. "Should I call back later when you have time to sort out your loss?"

"No. Tell me about her now."

"She had been ill for some months, under medication. But she constantly overdid with the children."

"Children?" Sydney gasped. "Miss Broderick had children?"

"Six of them."

"If she had children, why on earth am I her sole heir?"

For the first time he seemed amused. "It would seem for the time being that you have inherited the children as well."

A piece of land and six children! "How old are they?"

She heard him shuffling through papers again. "The oldest is nine, the youngest three. When Miss Broderick had her last heart attack, we tried to persuade her to go to the hospital. She refused because of the children. . . . As her lawyer, I am responsible for placing them. . . . Are you still with me, Miss Barrington?"

"Of course."

"They're not *her* children. She was their caregiver. We will have to place them. Perhaps you wish to be consulted on this?"

She hadn't spent much time with children except for visiting those in the hospital ward. She liked children—liked their quaint way of speaking, their funny little sayings, their innocence. But whatever would she do with six of them?

Gallagher's dispassionate voice turned edgy as he asked for directions on the disposal of Abigail's remains. "As her sole heir, we need to know your pleasure."

"What is your usual custom?"

"Quite like your own. Her will calls for immediate burial in St. Michael's Cemetery. Should I go ahead with plans?"

Of course. She had no desire to arrange another funeral. But he staved off her response when he said, "We are aware that you have a corporation to run. Your father's business."

How does he know that? she wondered.

"So there is no need for you to come," he continued. "I will be happy to act on your behalf. Sell the property—transfer the funds to you as soon as they are available. Dispose of the children. I already have a buyer in mind. I'll just send you the paperwork authorizing me—"

"A buyer for the children?"

He chuckled without humor. "The property, Miss Barrington."

No, she thought, irritated by Gallagher's brusque manner. *I will not authorize you to make decisions on my behalf. This woman could have been a flesh and blood relative. And I will not let you dispose of children as though they were rusty garden tools.*

She realized as she spoke heatedly with the man that it was not the CEO of Barrington sitting here engaged in a conversation across the world, but Millicent Barrington's offspring, ready to fight on behalf of hurting children. The thought pleased her.

Her attention was diverted momentarily to the river and her longing to get away from Randolph. But how could she think of using the death of a woman in a Cotswold village in England as an escape? Still, she said, "Mr. Gallagher, I must speak to my lawyers here. If possible, I will arrange my schedule to travel to England. I have business matters in Europe quite frequently. It will simply be a matter of adjusting my schedule."

"So you can attend the funeral?" he asked curtly.

"No. For the settling of the will—the selling of any property. And, as you said, the disposing of the children—"

Instead of static, there seemed to be silence. She imagined him covering the mouthpiece, seeking the opinion of someone else. Then he was back. "Your coming to England won't be necessary."

"But it will, Mr. Gallagher. I can't just let Miss Broderick's passing go unnoticed. You are obviously experienced at selling property—but we will not sell the children."

She heard him suck in his breath and decided that he was displeased with her decision. She didn't like what was happening on the other end of the world, but whoever this Abigail Broderick had been, perhaps she needed a friend to settle her affairs.

Sydney could spare a week or two, longer if necessary. Another inspection of the shipyard on the Tyne would be a good excuse for traveling abroad. And a dinner invitation to the manager of the carrier project would be a good investment of her time, especially if she selected one of the elegant restaurants in London. Calculating quickly, she knew she could arrange to leave within days. A week at most.

She grabbed a scrap of paper from her pocket. "Let me have a number where I can reach you, Mr. Gallagher." She jotted down his London number. "And your Cotswold listing? . . . Now, tell me, who is caring for the children at this time?"

His answer seemed indefinite, flustered. "A Mrs. Quigley. But there is no way to talk directly with her."

There is a way, Sydney thought, *but you don't want me to contact her.* "We'll be in touch, Mr. Gallagher. Perhaps we should meet in your London office."

"Yes . . . of course."

"We'll arrange that when I call back."

Suddenly she had the upper hand and knew it. Whatever was going on in Edmund Gallagher's mind, she had put him on the defensive. "You said the children were in the Cotswolds. In Stow-on-the-Woodland, wasn't it?"

"I didn't say, but that is where they are. But, Miss Barrington, they are in good hands. Trust me."

That's the one thing I won't do, she thought.

She hung up the phone and stared across at the sunlit waterfall. The tumultuous waters raged over the rock cliff and tumbled down in an ear-splitting force, and yet she felt an unbelievable calm. A peace. She should be overwhelmed, confused. And she was. But across the ocean she had just inherited a piece of land and six children. Tomorrow she would make the final decision on whether to pack, close up the house, and fly to England—to a solicitor who might not delight in her arrival. And to her new responsibility—six young children who needed permanent lodging.

Eight

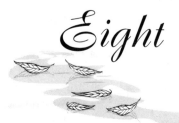

In London Edmund Gallagher slammed his knuckled fist on his desk and glared at the younger man sitting across from him. "It didn't go the way I expected, Marshall," he said.

"How did you expect it to go?"

"I thought Miss Barrington would allow me to handle the legal matters on this end—without her coming here."

"You lied to her. How long do you think you can deceive her into believing that Abigail Broderick is dead?"

Edmund rubbed his bruised knuckles. "My partners forced my hand. They knew Broderick was critical, and then yesterday I rushed things when I told them she was dead." He mopped his brow. "They knew the contents of her will. Rentley told me to get on the line and notify Miss Barrington. If I hadn't called her, Rentley or Blackstone would have. Blackstone is nervous enough about the problems we face when Jonas Willoughby discovers he's not the heir to Broadshire Manor."

He nursed his knuckles again. "I may still be able to persuade her that she is not needed on this end. She's talking to her own lawyers—that's a problem, but I'll work around it."

"Even if you persuade her to stay home, what happens when it comes time to hand over the property to her? You can't give away possessions when Abigail Broderick is still alive."

"You're the fool who said she was dying, Doctor."

Marshall escaped into a silence that infuriated Edmund. They had known each other all their lives, played on the Cotswold Hills, took their separate degrees in London. But they had never been close friends. Edmund at thirty-nine was the more ambitious man, well esteemed in the office of Gallagher, Blackstone, and Rentley. He had grown up near Bourton-on-the-Water, but he was a Londoner at heart— a serious-looking man with thick-rimmed glasses and curly brown hair prematurely peppered with gray, a man who rarely admitted to a sheep-grazing background. Marshall Wallis, a year younger, was content to live in the village, serving the people as a physician and spending his spare time fishing on the Windrush.

Although Edmund's firm headquartered in the heart of London, he still maintained his father's Cotswold office. He traveled to the Cotswolds two days a week with an eye to doubling profits, not from the country folk but from the growing populace of Londoners setting up holiday homes in Gloucestershire. The Broadshire property represented his ticket to independent wealth. Once he turned the manor into a hotel, it would open Stow-on-the-Woodland to tourism, a venture that would draw hundreds of tourists away from Bourton-on-the-Water.

Marshall rubbed his brow. "You've opened one of those kettles of worms, Edmund. The woman expects an inheritance now."

"I'll tell her that Abigail left heavy debts—that we must sell the estate to pay them off. I'll borrow funds from the firm—juggle a few major accounts to compensate Miss Barrington with a token amount of money. It's not as though she were a relative."

"Your partners will let you get by with that?"

"My partners will never know the money was missing. Once I take over Broadshire Manor, I'll pay them back. I'll sell portions of the property to developers. I'm not an idiot,

Marshall. I don't intend to stay with Blackstone and Rentley all my life."

"You've gone too far this time. Deceiving Abigail or Miss Barrington is one thing—fraud within your firm is another. And I'll have no part of it."

"You have no choice. It's cooperate with me or I will destroy you. Your wife would not like that."

Marshall winced. "Keep my wife out of this. Once the people of Stow-on-the-Woodland get wind of what you're doing, they will run you out of town—if your firm doesn't send you to prison before that."

"You would like that, wouldn't you?"

"Your plans will fail, Edmund. Blackstone and Rentley started the firm long before they took you in as a partner."

"Your point?"

"They made a mistake taking you in."

"I was top in my class. High levels."

"But not an intelligent man. They'll realize that someday. Are you aware that Jonas Willoughby is home now?"

"Yes. He made two appointments with me to discuss selling the property and the legal ramifications of placing his father in a permanent residence. I promised to find him a buyer for the property. But I must put him off as long as Abigail is alive."

"Then he doesn't know that Barrington is the sole heir?"

"What difference does it make? Jonas plans to go back to sea. I'm biding my moves accordingly. Once he's gone, I would have no difficulty persuading Abigail to sell me the property—if she lives long enough to make that decision."

"I don't want to see you go down, Edmund, but if you try to take over the manor illegally, I'll stop you."

"How, Marshall? I have the law on my side and the power to ruin you. Where would the village be without a health center? Tell me—just how long does Abigail have? Days? Weeks? Hours?"

Marshall said quietly, "I have no idea. But I'd be glad if the old girl lived forever—and put a stop to your madness."

Sydney awakened to a thick smog hemming the city in and thought at once of the strangers in the Cotswolds who had stepped uninvited into her life. For the first time since taking over Barrington Enterprises, she decided to work at home. Alone. She needed time to think about Abigail Broderick. Something hovered on the edge of memory, some link to this stranger who had died.

Before showering, she browsed the Internet, plugging in names and places in the Cotswolds. She found only one small segment about Stow-on-the-Woodland:

A quaint Cotswold hamlet along the River Windrush, fifteen miles from Bourton-on-the-Water. Noted for its fifteenth-century St. Michael's Cathedral, a historical water mill, and its trout streams.

Her fingers flew over the keys in search of places to stay in Bourton-on-the-Water. She found hotels and inns in the center of town. The names *Mousetrap* and *Old Manse Hotel* intrigued her, but she booked her room at The Sheepfold, a bed-and-breakfast along the Windrush. She pictured herself wandering through peaceful English gardens and traipsing the footpaths into the countryside, or hiking along the streams in the village where Abigail Broderick had lived and died. Peaceful? What was she thinking? Six children would be dogging her footsteps.

Her excitement built as she turned her search engine to people. Abigail Broderick's name did not appear on the screen. But she found a listing for Edmund Gallagher: *Edmund Gallagher of Gallagher, Blackstone, and Rentley, solicitors, London, England.*

Would it please him if she called to tell him that she was flying to Stow-on-the-Woodland within the week? An hour passed. Two. Finally, she stretched her aching shoulders and knew that she needed the rushing sound of water to help her make a decision.

Forty minutes later, she stood on a narrow stretch of beach overlooking Puget Sound, listening to the waves pounding relentlessly against the ferry dock. The wind caught the breaking rollers and swept them toward her, spraying her face. The thick swirling mist that obliterated the city at dawn had blown out to sea. Still the weather remained overcast, leaving the sky and the water a dismal gray. Sand particles blew into her eyes as she walked toward the picnic benches. The sounds that surrounded her intruded on her thoughts about the unknown stranger who had left her everything— all of her possessions and six children.

Would going to England be Sydney's folly? Something for her board of directors and Randolph to gloat over, laugh about? Gallagher could settle everything without her presence. But again as a gentle wave washed ashore, she knew that she did not trust the British solicitor. She felt certain that he did not have the best interest of these children at heart.

As seagulls skimmed across the surface of the water, other hikers jogged toward her, their voices in muffled undertones. Above came the noise of a helicopter; on the road to her left, the cranky overdrive of a battered truck on the street. Her sneakers beat a rhythmic tread to the blast of the ferry whistle and the creaking of the boat slipping from the pier.

Sydney plunged her hands into her pockets and plowed on until she came to a disposal unit, framed by a stone wall. Leaning against the wall, she tried to picture the faces of the children in the Cotswolds and could not, but she would pack toys and one or two of her mother's dolls for the trip to England.

Taking her cell phone from her jacket, she plugged in Randolph's number at the office. "Randolph, this is Sydney."

"I've been calling everyone. Your neighbors. Your caretaker at the cabin. Where have you been?" he exploded.

"I'm all right. I just needed time to think."

"About us?"

"No. I've been walking. Making plans for a trip abroad."

Hopefully, he said, "Really? Do the plans include me?"

"Not this time, Randy. I'm planning a trip alone."

"You'd better think about the work piling up on your desk."

Her thoughts winged to her father's upholstered chair and ottoman where he had read to her so long ago from *The Old Man and the Sea* and from his favorite, *For Whom the Bell Tolls*. Aaron was in many ways like Hemingway—popular, tough, scornful of other men's ideas. He loved Hemingway, but thankfully her father had not been there to scorn the toll of the church bell calling his friends and employees to his own funeral.

Randolph broke into her thoughts. "Sydney, you're not hearing a word I'm saying. What's that roar in the background?"

"The breakers. The ferries. I'm down at the beach."

It set him off again. "Barrington Enterprises is your responsibility. Have you checked on Wall Street this morning?"

"No, and I didn't have coffee either. They usually go hand-in-hand." This morning she hadn't thought about the ticker tape that charted the all-consuming rise and fall of her investments.

"Stock prices are down, Syd. Interest rates rising."

"Stop fussing. Our business is booming. What more do you want?"

"If I were in charge," he snarled, "I would be at my desk right now signing those new government contracts, not out walking on the beach."

"We'll talk about the contracts tomorrow."

"You're not coming in this afternoon? Great! Daron Emery has points on the carrier project to discuss with you. And your secretary has fielded your calls all day. And those defense contracts for the plant in Tennessee need your signature, not mine," he reminded her.

"That's going to change in the next few weeks. I'm leaving you in charge when I'm gone. That's what you've been wanting all along, isn't it? A chance to run Barrington?"

Her words got through to him. "You're not running out on me? It's not that quarrel the other day?"

"The other day is history."

His voice grew thick, throaty. "Am I too?"

"We'll talk about that later. I want you to set up a meeting with the board of directors first thing in the morning. We'll discuss us—my plans for you then."

"In a room full of executives? Surely, I deserve more than that."

You deserve so much more, she thought. "Don't worry, Randolph. I won't embarrass you in front of our colleagues. Making a good impression is too important to both of us."

She stretched her long legs in front of her, raking the sand with her shoe. "But I've learned something. A good impression is only temporary. It doesn't make for lasting happiness."

"Oh, no. We're back to your finding your Shangri-La again. You can't fly off on some harebrained holiday, hunting for something you'll never find. Where are you going?"

She considered telling him about the children in the Cotswolds, but would he understand? He had made it clear often enough. When he married, he did not want children. The best thing she could do for both of them was go away.

"I'm going to Europe."

"Europe? Is there more trouble with the shipyard?"

"No. I'll explain everything tomorrow."

He cleared his throat. "Sydney, I must see you. Go back to the house and I'll pick you up for a late lunch."

"Not today. I'll see you in the morning."

"Then have dinner with me?"

"Not tonight. I have to go now. It's windy down here."

She disconnected before he could argue with her and began walking back to the car. Why did he stir such mixed emotions in her? She liked him, disliked him. Cared about him, avoided him. But he was right. Barrington Enterprises with its billions invested in defense projects was her responsibility. How could she think about England when she had Aaron Barrington's empire to run?

Above her the overcast sky had lifted; billowy white clouds had blown in. Sydney came out of her own foggy mist, her decision made. No matter what Randolph thought, she must fly to England.

Nine

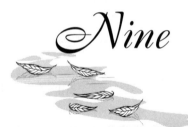

Sydney needed legal advice, but not from her corporate lawyers or by pulling a name from the yellow pages. She wanted Jeffrey VanBurien. At the thought of him, she pictured his features vividly. Tall and blade-thin. Long-legged. Fair-haired, with a thick blond mustache that looked good on him and sharp blue eyes that glinted when he smiled.

She reached for her phone, dialed his number in Chicago, and waited for his secretary to put her through to Jeffrey. She had been exhausted and hungry when she met him at a business conference in Chicago, shortly after her parents' plane crash. The hotel dining room had been too full to seat her immediately.

"Ah! Stranded in the Windy City and hungry!" said a voice behind her. "Why don't we find another place to eat?"

She had turned and looked up into the bluest of eyes. "Sorry, I don't go running around the streets of Chicago with a stranger. My fiancé wouldn't approve."

He lifted her hand and checked the diamond. "My luck. So we'll have to eat here."

When he produced his business card, she said, "Oh, you're a lawyer."

"Jeffrey VanBurien at your service."

"I could use a good lawyer, an honest one preferably."

The blue eyes danced. "I am good. Even my brother hires me as his personal defender. And I can be honest, if I have to."

He beckoned to the maitre d'. "We were told there's an hour's wait. We don't have an hour. The lady is hungry now. Perhaps you would be so good as to get the management and tell him Celeste VanBurien's son is here with a guest."

He was back within minutes. "This way, sir."

During dinner, he had told her about himself—born in Chicago, a mother well-known in Oak Park, his father dead and buried in Alabama.

When she confided her fears at taking over her father's business, he had encouraged her and offered his help.

On the spot, she had retained him for off-the-cuff advice. It had been a good move on her part, one that mushroomed into a warm friendship. Jeff was like having a big brother to lean on, a broad shoulder to cry on, a trustworthy confidant that she could phone on a moment's notice. Whenever she changed planes in Chicago—and that was often enough—he'd be there, waiting for her with a big grin and a thermos full of coffee or a box of candy.

Now she twisted the telephone cord on her fingers as she waited for him to answer and smiled as he said, "Jeff Van-Burien speaking."

She remembered his pleasant, laughing voice. "Jeff, it's Sydney Barrington. What took you so long to answer?"

"A rich client. How are you? Been weeks since I heard from you. Are you beautiful as ever?"

She glanced down at her faded jeans and brushed back her gnarled hair, windblown from the beach. "Not exactly. But I need a favor."

"You're paying me retainer's fees. Shoot."

"I'm flying to England on Wednesday. I may be running into legal problems."

"With the airline?"

"No, with a British solicitor."

"Run that one by me again."

"According to this lawyer, a woman by the name of Abigail Broderick just died and left her inheritance to me."

"That I should be so lucky. Did she leave you a mansion?"

"Don't joke, Jeff. I'm pressed for time."

"Sorry; I guess I didn't know you had rich friends in far-away places. So what's up with this Abigail Broderick?"

"It's the lawyer who's troubling me. I have this uncanny feeling that he can't be trusted."

"A lot of people evaluate lawyers that way." He became more professional now. "I can't judge uncanny feelings. Is he fraudulent? Has he let you down before?"

"I haven't met him. We've just talked by phone. But there's land and children to worry about. He wanted to send me some papers to sign so he could settle everything without my being there. Said he already had a buyer for the property."

She pictured Jeff leaning forward, his elbows propped on his desk. "Don't sign a thing. When did this Miss Broderick die?"

"She isn't buried yet. I know that."

"You sound like you don't know much about her."

"I don't even know if we've met. But six children are involved, and the lawyer plans to dispose of them. At least that's the way he described it."

"Syd, if you think he's a hoax, why go over there?"

"I have legitimate reasons for checking on our European facilities. In the last eighteen months, since Mom and Dad's plane crash, I've been sending others to do my job. It's time for me to go myself."

"But you're still afraid of flying—and you're going on another overseas flight?"

"I have to for the sake of those children."

He whistled. "You always were a sucker for kids. I think you better tell me everything. And start from the beginning."

"The lawyer's name is Edmund Gallagher. I think he's anxious to sell the property before I get there." She filled in the rest of the details, choking up as she spoke of the children.

While she composed herself, he said, "Sydney, we could get married and raise those kids together. You'd have to live in Chicago, of course. And maybe you'd have to work part-time so we could support them."

For some reason his nonsense brought on a flood of tears. The crazy galoot would probably do it. "That's the sweetest offer I've had all day, but I'd rather have you as my lawyer," she said.

"Just my luck. So what steps have you taken?"

"I've made my reservation with a brief layover in New York." She gave him the flight numbers and departure time.

"Too bad you aren't transferring in Chicago. We could have dinner together. Syd, you're okay about flying over the ocean?"

"I'm trying not to think about it. And I have a meeting with my board of directors in the morning. I'll drop my bombshell then. I'm leaving Randolph Iverson in charge."

"Your call. Anything else I should know?"

"You have my arrival time in London. I'll rent a car at Heathrow. I booked a room at The Sheepfold—a bed-and-breakfast in Bourton-on-the-Water. From there, it's an easy drive to Stow-on-the-Woodland. Fifteen miles or so."

"Don't do anything rash. Just meet with Mr. Gallagher and hear what he has to say."

"I plan to look over my own inheritance."

"Look, but stay out of trouble. And we have a major problem, Syd. I'm not qualified for British law." His words sounded muffled now, and she wondered whether he was rubbing his mustache or chewing the tip of his pen.

"I understand that, but I trust your advice."

"I'll browse in my law books the minute we hang up. Don't worry, Sydney. You said you're staying at The Sheepfold in Bourton-on-the-Water? I'll contact you there." More lightly, he asked, "How's lover boy?"

"Randolph? We're not engaged any longer."

"Sorry about that." He didn't sound sorry at all.

"Jeff, all I've done is talk about me. How are you?"

"Been putting my life back together. Do you remember me telling you about my half-brother, Chandler Reynolds?"

"The music critic who works for American Intelligence?"

"The CIA is a sideline, and if he ever gets in trouble, Langley won't know him."

"What about him?"

"He's in England where you want to be. Married now. I'll fax you his number. And, Sydney, we finally decided to have that get-together. I'm taking six weeks off from the firm and flying to London myself. We're going to give this brother thing a shot."

"Then you'll be in England?"

"And we'll be in touch. It's cutting it tight, but I'll see about changing my booking and flying with you."

"Oh, you don't have to do that."

"I know. But I'd hate to miss the opportunity of traveling with a beautiful woman."

She sensed he was about to hang up. "Jeff, thanks so much."

"No problem. My legal fees come high."

"I know. Just bill Barrington Enterprises."

"I'll do that," he said cheerfully and hung up.

Sydney stood at the door of the conference room and surveyed the thirteen directors at the oval table. They sat rigidly, as stiff as the backs of their maroon leather chairs. Bespeckled Sam Rosman twiddled his thumbs. Max Berger twisted his tie. Randolph sat beside him—immaculate as always, his business savvy apparent in the cut of his dark suit and silk tie.

She caught Randolph's eye as she entered. He who was always confident, always putting forth his best front, looked wary. He stood as she reached the head of the table. For a moment she feared he would brazenly brush a kiss across her cheek.

He slid the chair in behind her. "Are you all right, Syd?"

Ignoring his concern, she rested her wrists on the table and said, "Good morning, everyone."

Eighteen months before, it would have been, "Good morning, gentlemen."

Her father had excluded women on his executive board. In her first three months as CEO, Sydney had fired one man and replaced him with capable Ivy Meckerton. Another of her father's old cronies had died six months into her takeover. Against strong opposition, she clung to a small clause in the company policy—her father's safeguard for his own leadership—and assumed the right to choose her own replacements: another woman, three years her junior. The younger woman sat with her tapered fingers locked, her gaze straying toward Randolph.

The directors were an intelligent lot, and if they weren't loyal to her, they were loyal to the memory of her dad. Financially secure, they weren't apt to leave Barrington Enterprises, even with Sydney at the helm. Though some of them still struggled with a little girl image, they respected her business aplomb, her drive. The original dip in profits at the death of her dad had long since surged upward. Barrington Enterprises still held its firm grip in the world market.

Sydney planned to say something that would infuriate them all—but again policy gave her the right to do so. "I'm leaving town for a while on a brief business holiday to England," she announced. She glanced at Randolph, her gaze steadfast. "Mr. Iverson will be in charge while I'm away."

Max Berger quit twisting his tie, his sleepy gaze alert now. "Sydney, your father always left me in charge."

And I never understood why.

She made a mental note to offer Berger a sizable retirement package on her return, one that would allow him a graceful withdrawal and eliminate the slowdown that was obviously taking place. Max was a good man, but he should have taken his social security and pension three years ago and not hung on as the oldest member of the board. She would never fire him. She had sat on his knee as a child and delighted in the dolls and boxes of candy he had given her over the years.

"Max, Randolph will keep you apprised of what's going on."

Ivy Meckerton looked puzzled. "That trip was scheduled for next month. I thought I was handling that for you."

"Next time, Ivy. I want to see firsthand how things are going in our European divisions."

"But I know you dislike flying since—"

Sydney smiled gratefully at Ivy.

Randolph came out of his silence. "Foreign negotiations?" he said scathingly. "I usually handle those."

"Not this time."

He nodded to the others, his eyes unsmiling. "It would seem that Miss Barrington has already made the decision to go herself." *Without consulting me,* his voice seemed to say.

"Trust me, Mr. Iverson. This is best for all of us. I have a private matter to tend to as well. I've just been advised of the death of a—friend."

Ivy leaned forward. "We're so sorry. But will you be all right flying alone? I could go with you."

"Randolph will need your help." *Your wisdom,* she thought.

A lump rose in Sydney's throat as she thought of her dad's last time at the conference table—making arrangements, handing out assignments. A handsome, silver-haired gentleman, a man who lived to make money, building success upon success. He had left the conference room and the next day flown off with his wife, not to their intended destination in Europe, but into eternity.

Sydney had flown across country several times since then, always with a knot in her stomach. But she had not flown out over the ocean since that crash off the waters of Long Island. She blinked, remembering that miserable moment when she had looked out on the bobbing pieces of the aircraft caught in the stormy swells of the water. She had turned away, tears burning behind her eyes. Her stomach tightened even now.

"I'll be all right, Ivy." She flashed her confident, executive smile. The no-nonsense, no questions asked variety. "Now, regarding those government contracts from Washington—"

As the room emptied, Randolph caught her hand. "You're running away."

"From you?"

"From life."

She pulled away from him and gathered up her papers. "I can afford to do anything I like."

"Stay. We'll work it out. We can send Ivy in your place."

"Randolph, someone really did die."

He licked his thin lips. "A close friend?"

"An older woman. I didn't know about her until—"

She couldn't speak with the lump in her throat. Why was she trying to explain the unexplainable to Randolph? She didn't even understand her own sense of loss.

"You have a business to run here."

"You can handle it. You know the company better than I do."

"Aren't you afraid I'll take control while you're gone and change everything your father wanted?"

"You're too honest, Randolph. Too loyal."

"You don't believe that for a minute."

"Then you're forgetting the board of directors and the company lawyers who will make certain everything runs smoothly. It's up to you. I thought you would like handling things while I'm gone. Running things—isn't that what you've always wanted?"

"What I want is to be with you. I just wish your father would stop coming between us."

"I don't understand why you dislike him so."

"Because you are so much like him. Assertive. Ambitious."

"It takes that to run this corporation."

"I wish you would just give all of this up and marry me."

"Cunning man that you are. Then you could take the helm of the ship permanently, is that it?"   .

95

"Your father promised it to me."

"No, he trained you for leadership, but he never promised that you would take over his job."

"Then delegate more of your responsibilities to me."

"I just did here at this conference table. Weren't you listening? I put you in charge while I'm gone."

"Syd, do you plan to check up on my last trips to Europe to find out whether I did everything according to Aaron's wishes? Someday, you're going to wake up. Your father never did anything that didn't benefit himself."

He flipped the end of his tie. Smoothed it out again. "I'm the first one to admit that I wouldn't be where I am today without him, but he molded me to fit his own schemes. I think, my dear Sydney, he did the same for you."

"You're wrong. My father was a good man. A hard worker. He was kind to those who worked for him."

"He was more Greek myth than kindly. He was Icarian by nature, like a Greek god. But I think he flew too high with some of his bidding. And I think he had his wings clipped with that shipyard project. Someday you're going to discover another side to the man you adored, and your father's going to come tumbling down from his ivory tower. We're still trying to track down a couple of his accounts. The Broadshire account for one."

Her brows puckered at the word.

"The account records amounts of money transferred to a Swiss bank. Nothing else. No addresses. That's poor management, Syd. And the Swiss bank is tight-lipped about the recipient. Periodic transfers. In varied amounts. Was that one of your father's defense projects? Or another of his follies?"

"Stop it, Randy. My father was the most honest man I know."

"Really?" He sighed. "You're right. But he was not always fair with other men's dreams."

"Yours, for instance?" she asked gently.

"I worked closely with your father. I saw the darker side. He never let another man's dreams stand in the way of his own. He was ambitious, forceful, scheming."

Like you, she thought.

"He was good at what he did. Never forget, Dad built this corporation from scratch."

"By exploiting his competitors."

"If you found him so despicable, why didn't you resign long ago?"

"Because I wanted to be near you."

She shrugged. "Randy, I feel sorry for you."

For a second she considered putting him on the streets to find his own way to the top. But she needed him at Barrington Enterprises. Sydney felt her smile coming back. He did have a handsome face, but his eyes proved his best feature—seductive, dewy-eyed, yet sad now as he looked at her. She went over to him and touched her finger to his lips. "Let's not quarrel. Not now. We need some time apart. I think all of this is just about the two of us. I don't think it has anything to do with my father."

He pressed her fingers against his mouth and kissed them. "Don't go. Stay. Marry me."

"Dear Randolph, I'll never change. I'll always be ambitious, as you call it. I think what you want is an ordinary cog in the wheel for your life's companion. A wife who will stand behind her husband and say nothing."

She started for the door of the conference room. He blocked her way. "Promise me you'll come back."

"Why wouldn't I?"

"Because deep inside, you're searching for something and I don't think I'm part of that plan."

When they reached her private office, she wondered whether she was doing the right thing. She turned and found herself inches from him, close to that familiar scent he always wore. With her mind's eye she traced his features. Remembered the warmth of his arms. She reached out again and touched his cheek, regretting the bitter quarrel that still stood between them.

"My return ticket is open-ended."

"That's forever."

Her hand slipped back to her side. "I'm sorry, Randolph."

"Sydney, I want to be with you. Let me go home with you tonight? I'll drive you to the airport in the morning."

"No, that's not a good idea. And I'm not leaving until Wednesday. I've already ordered an airport limousine."

"You could cancel the limousine."

When she looked into his eyes again, her anger at him melted completely. He needed her, but she slipped behind her desk to separate them. She was sailing dangerously close to thin ice. Her skin prickled. The knot in her stomach doubled. She could almost taste her loneliness. What was wrong with surrendering to Randy's charms? Wasn't that what they both wanted? Wasn't that the way to put aside their quarrel?

Purposefully, she cleared her desk. The silence dragged.

"Sydney, look at me."

She glanced up. He stood with his hands in his pockets, his face so familiar—so much a part of her life—that it seemed impossible to remember when their friendship had really begun.

"I'm afraid I'm losing you," he said sadly.

"You lost me last week." She didn't add, *But then, I was never really yours.*

His tone, rancorous moments ago, was whipped, defeated. "I need you. Let me stay tonight? We can work things out."

Don't say another word, she thought. *Just go. Go on your own, because I might not have the strength to send you away again.*

He held her gaze, his eyes grave, mirthless, the glimmer of hope fading. She had let him down, throttled him; her leaving was the last thing he expected. She wanted to say she was truly sorry.

98

Sorry for him. Sorry for what might have been. But the die was cast. She was being drawn to the Cotswolds in a way she could neither understand nor explain.

He took a step toward her. His eyes said it all. *You're dazzling, beautiful, love of my life.* But where was the chemistry between them? How long could she go on pretending?

"Sydney, I need you. I love you."

"Please," she said. "Please go."

Ten

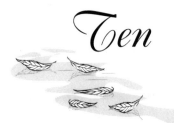

Northwood Headquarters, a highly classified area, crawled with gold braid. Driving in through the security gate, Jonas stepped back into his own world, a man's world for the most part. NATO commands from several countries found posting here: the Americans and Dutch, French and Italians, the Greeks. Lunch in the wardroom allowed him to keep his language skills current. He could switch easily into German, French, or Spanish.

Minutes later, he stood outside Captain McIntyre's office, grinning to himself as he touched the three gold stripes on his uniform sleeve. As the clerk admitted him, McIntyre extended his hand across an uncluttered desk. Jonas had only seconds to survey the Spartan room. Everything looked shipshape, like quarters on board the carrier. The only personal touch in the room was the large ship's model on the captain's desk.

"Your model looks like one of the frigates from the Falklands, sir. The *Ardent* or the *Antelope?*"

"One just like them. The *Brownlee*. It was my first ship. Your father was C.O. then. Come, I have pictures over here."

Jonas steeled his shoulders and plunged in. "Sir, I would appreciate compassionate leave for a few days."

"Good grief, Willoughby. Did the Admiral die and we haven't been informed?"

"No, sir. But the friend who takes care of him is not well."

McIntyre dismissed the request, saying, "Commander, you know compassionate leave is for immediate family only. Now, come along, have a look at these old ships."

I worded it wrong, Jonas thought.

He tried again, but McIntyre led him to the far wall filled with photographs of ships that had sailed under Her Majesty's Service. His broad finger centered on the edge of one, straightening it. "This is the way the *Brownlee* looked the day I boarded her back in the Falklands. During one lull in the battle at San Carlos, your father went down to the injured and walked straight over to a dying midshipman. A lad about seventeen."

McIntyre clicked his tongue. "What a commanding officer. He came in with his cap crooked under one arm, his hair thick and black like yours, Willoughby. He took off his jacket, sat down, and took that young man's hand in his own."

The muscle in Jonas's neck grew taut. *He never held my hand,* he thought. *Ever.* His father had called it too unprofessional, too unpolished for a senior rank. *Be a man, Jonas.*

"Your father called the lad by name. Said, 'Neil, I have a son about your age. I keep his picture on my desk.' You could hear the pride in his voice when he talked about you. Said you had gone to Gordonstoun and would go on to Dartmouth."

Jonas kept his gaze fixed on the picture of the ship, trying to see his father through McIntyre's eyes.

"He told Neil that you spent your holidays in Stow-on-the-Woodland, right along the Windrush. And quite bluntly, he asked, 'You're from that area, aren't you, Neil?'"

"I was in the next bunk, injured myself, and I saw Neil's eyes brim with tears at the mention of the countryside. 'Yes, sir. Gloucestershire. Winchcombe,' he said. For almost twenty minutes, your father talked to him about the Cotswold Hills. About sheep grazing and waterwheels spinning at the mill. Quite in the middle of everything your father said, 'Her Majesty is proud of you, son. Grateful for your sacrifice. You will be long remembered.'"

He squared another frame on the wall. "He made it a point to tell the boy he'd visit his parents the next time he went home on leave. He didn't tell him he was dying, but the boy knew. And I knew, and I was frightened for him. Then your father's conversation flowed quite simply into a description of heaven."

Jonas cleared his throat. "And did he tell him how to get there?"

"You would have thought he'd been there himself speaking of the river of life and golden streams and a pain-free existence."

To Jonas, the man that McIntyre described seemed vastly different from the man he knew. He couldn't imagine his father sitting beside a dying man. The Admiral hadn't even come home for his wife's funeral. No, that wasn't fair. His father's ship was in the Far East on a crisis posting, too far away to bury the woman he loved.

Jonas's gaze slid along to other ships. A big battlewagon. A World War II submarine. The *Cavalier*, in dry dock now. He ran his teeth over his lower lip. Both the *Cavalier* and his father had followed distinguished careers. Both had been retired to inactive status—a death warrant to both the ship and the Admiral.

Captain McIntyre demanded his attention again. "Your father stayed with Neil until he died and then he stood up, tall and wiry like he is, and put his jacket on and squared his visored cap and I knew as they pulled the curtain around that boy, I would gladly follow your father into battle whenever, wherever. I did—twice on other ships. We never spoke of that incident in the Falklands, but he had my undying respect."

He faced Jonas. "I consider your father a great man. He deserved to be an admiral. To serve with the Admiralty. And now I have the opportunity to work with his son."

"So I'm here because of my father?"

"It influenced me, but your record is good, Willoughby."
He pointed to the *HMS Invincible*. "Your last posting, wasn't
it?"

"Yes, a great ship."

McIntyre's jaw tensed. "I can't say I favor the changes
coming in the *Andrew*—this man's Navy won't be the same.
With the reduction of ships, promotions will be hard to
come by. I'm still adjusting to a combined air fleet. Can you
believe it? The RN and RAF joining forces. Your father left
at a good time."

"I'll miss the rivalry between the two services. But flying
never appealed to my father."

"Is that why you chose it, Willoughby?" Wisely, he didn't
wait for the answer. "Tell me, how is the old man? I've been
meaning to get over to see him."

"He'd like that. He'd welcome your visit, but it's not likely
he'll remember you."

"But he'd remember his ships."

"That he would, sir. It's all he talks about. Shouting orders from his bed. Telling us to clear the harbor at Portsmouth so we can set sail. Yes, he'd remember the ships."

"And does he remember you, Jonas?"

"Not when I first got back. But he does now."

"I'm sorry that your father's health is failing. Is that why
you transferred to Northwood? A bloody shame, that's what
I call it. Your not taking your own command. But the *Invincible* is due back in Portsmouth in September. By jove, it
would be splendid if you were ready to board her again."

"It depends on my father—"

"He'd never stand in your way of a promotion. Why you
gave up that ship, I'll never understand. It must have shocked
him too. But it must comfort you, Willoughby, knowing
your father has always been proud of you. He constantly
bragged about you as you came up through the ranks."

"I wish he had told me how proud he was."

If the captain was surprised, he masked it. "Perhaps you weren't listening."

He walked back to his desk, Jonas following. "Sir, I keep hoping I'll be offered another command when things settle down."

"The best you can hope for is to go back to flying. You'd better not delay too long. Another two years and the French Dassault Rafale or the Eurofighters will replace the Harriers."

"I'd like to fly the Eurofighter—and be on hand for the maiden voyage of one of the new carriers."

The captain browsed through the folder in front of him. "Squadron commander. Naval duty in the Adriatic. On Northern Ireland patrol. Twice to the Gulf. You spoiled your record turning down the command of a minehunter. It didn't sit well with the Admiralty."

Jonas ran his teeth over his lower lip again. His father had drummed the ground rules into him. "Never forget, Jonas, an officer is married to the Service. You marry the Navy."

McIntyre continued. "The Navy always cares for its own, Willoughby. Even in the Admiral's condition, he would be provided for throughout his lifetime. They have a great residence in South Devon. Why don't you look into it?"

He didn't have the heart to say, "I did." Nor the courage to admit that he didn't have the stomach to turn his dad out to pasture. Instead he said, "I was surprised when they let my promotion go through."

"I argued on your behalf, Commander. Besides, I had a job for you here at Northwood, no matter how tentative. So you got the promotion. And I got the man." He smiled wryly. "Once I explain, you will understand why a compassionate leave is out."

He stretched his watchband. "I'm heading up an Irish project that should interest you. We're running against the clock with the IRA. Most favor peace, but we must ward off any factional groups trying last minute tactical maneuvers to ruin the fragile peace efforts." His gaze held steady. "I know about your fiancée. You have my sympathy. But to work with me, you must put aside any anger that you still hold against the IRA."

Jonas rubbed his chin with the back of his hand, staving off the sudden throbbing along his jaw.

"Sit down, Willoughby. I'll tell you what I have in mind."

With care, he detailed his own involvement in the Irish peace process as a military advisor, the need to track any active IRA members still hiding out in England, and the urgency to prevent any unprovoked attacks on British soil. "I don't have to tell you that resuming any IRA bombings would threaten the peace efforts and be a threat to Her Majesty's ships in Irish waters."

He smiled. "For the record, you are still working under NATO Intelligence. But for the next few weeks, you will be working directly under me. And, Willoughby, I will not tolerate a man working against me, seeking his own revenge."

McIntyre was questioning his loyalty? He said, "Have I stepped out of line somewhere, sir?"

"You tell me. With your transfer to Northwood, you're being vetted, checked out once again. Mostly at my request. If we are to work together, I demand your utmost loyalty, regardless of the personal cost to you."

Jonas nodded. "You still have reservations about me?"

"Your decision to turn down the command came at an odd time, Commander. Your father has been sick for months—and suddenly at the exact time when reports were coming to us about an Irish agent in the Cotswolds, your request for transfer came in."

"What would an IRA rebel be doing in Stow-on-the-Woodland?"

"I had intended to ask *you* that, Commander."

The muscles in Jonas's neck drew his features into a scowl. He could no more prevent it than he could his father's illness. But an Irish faction in the Cotswolds where sheep grazed peacefully and children played by the Windrush? Ludicrous. Stow-on-the-Woodland was not a town for trouble. He braced himself in the chair across from McIntyre. "Days ago, the vicar suggested the possibility of Irish problems in the village."

"But you didn't see fit to report that rumor to me?"

"The truth is, I didn't believe him. Why would I? I've known the people in the village all my life. I trust them."

"The MI5 report that reached my desk suggested the possibility of an IRA rebel hiding out in the woods near your home, Commander. Twenty-four hours later the revised report read 'wounded, still missing.' If he's still in your village, then someone has given him a place to hide."

Someone hiding a terrorist? The schoolmaster? The owner of Chutman's Pub? The parish priest? Abigail? No, not Abigail and not anyone at the manor. All of them were English to the core!

"Captain, a stranger was accidentally shot in our village the other evening. That may be the man you are talking about."

The crow's-foot lines by McIntyre's eyes deepened. "I hoped you would tell me about that. MI5's report also stated that you were in the village that night. But I find no report from you."

"Not much to tell. I heard the gunfire. There was an extensive search. I have no idea who he was or where he is now."

"But you came back to the base early. On Sunday, I believe. That's not your usual pattern, Willoughby. You usually wing in here just under the wire on Monday mornings. What happened?"

"Miss Broderick urged me to leave. She said it wouldn't sit well for the Admiral's son to be involved in a village shooting. Knowing the nature of my work here at Fleet Headquarters, I agreed. I packed and left at once."

"This Miss Broderick? Is she the Admiral's housekeeper?"

If I'm being vetted again, you already know she isn't.

106

He remained civil. "Griselda Quigley is the housekeeper. Abigail Broderick is more like a family member. She pretty much mothered me after my own mother died. It's hard to think of a time when Abigail wasn't there running the manor. In a way, she was always in charge. I'll never know how she talked my father into housing all those children, although my mother may have made that decision. She and Abigail were great friends. They often traveled together on the continent. I thought them inseparable."

"Housing what children, Willoughby?"

"Refugee children displaced by wars."

"A visionary. Was she too busy to marry?"

"She was engaged once to a British commando. He was killed in World War II. But she's still taking care of children."

"Would she harbor a wounded man with the children there?"

Did he make it? Abigail had asked. Abigail involved? Hiding someone? Urging Jonas to leave.

"I say, does this Miss Broderick have Irish ties?"

"Some Irish friends. Nothing more."

"Willoughby, any Brit caught aiding and abetting the IRA would be dealt with promptly. Any senior naval officer would face immediate dismissal. And probably be tried for treason."

"Sir, are you suggesting—"

"I am just reminding you of the severity of defending an Irish rebel, even if that rebel were a former classmate or a former boarder at Broadshire Manor. There can be no sympathy for the IRA in your village or anywhere else. The man may be wounded, but we are not dealing with some romantic freedom fighter. I trust that no one you know is embroiled in such a cause."

McIntyre leaned back in his chair. "Think about it, Willoughby. The person involved may be very close to you. Protecting an IRA terrorist means that person has lost his sense of loyalty to the Queen and the country."

Jonas felt as though Captain McIntyre saw him as the enemy. "Sir, we are on the same side."

"Good." The captain pulled a picture from the file and tossed it across the desk to Jonas. "Do you recognize this man?"

"Looks like it was taken in Belfast."

"I didn't ask for a location, Willoughby. Do you know him?"

He studied the side view of a young man caught unawares, standing on the hillside, his hair ruffled by a gust of wind. A wary countenance. A black-market rifle balanced over one shoulder. He stalled. "I'd have to see a close-up, Captain."

"What about this one?"

McIntyre tossed a color photo on top of the first. A gaunt, lifelike face loomed up at Jonas. Definitely, Conon O'Reilly's cold, steely eyes as green as a stormy sea. Fiery red hair. A face thinner than he remembered. A sense of déjà vu struck Jonas, a not unpleasant recollection warming him. "That's one of the lads from Gordonstoun when I was head boy. He was a superb soccer player. Gave all his classmates a run for their money."

"He's still running, Willoughby. He's an Irishman, one of the active IRA holding out on any peace agreement. Did this Miss Broderick of yours ever take in children from the IRA conflict?"

Something stirred inside Jonas. Conon O'Reilly, the crack shot on the rifle team at Gordonstoun. A rabble rouser politically. One of Abigail's boys that she wanted Jonas to look after. Louise flashed into his mind. In that instant, his war against Irish terrorism turned personally against this old school chum from Gordonstoun.

"That's Conon O'Reilly," he admitted. "I haven't seen him for years. He was one of Abigail Broderick's boys. He stayed at the manor for several months. Longer perhaps. Our paths didn't cross much after I left for Oxford and Dartmouth. But O'Reilly was a problem at the manor, a real troublemaker."

"Would that have made a difference to Miss Broderick?"

"She would never turn a child away—even one with a violent temper like O'Reilly had. He left when he was fourteen or fifteen. I don't think Abigail ever heard from him again."

McIntyre glanced out the window. "Did you know that Mr. O'Reilly's father was involved in the early years with the IRA? He was linked with the Warrenpoint bomb and Brighton five years later. A bloody man in the beginning. Did you ever meet him?"

"No, Conon's father was like mine. Neither of them made a habit of visiting Gordonstoun."

"Willoughby, about the time of the Good Friday Peace Agreement, the older O'Reilly switched loyalties—became a strong advocate for peace. Went pro-British. I served with him at the conference table, but his political betrayal didn't sit well with his old friends. Nor with his son. Someone murdered him en route to a meeting with the British Prime Minister."

"Another case of the hunter hunted down."

"Pathetic, really. He was killed in Belfast where he was born. Just when he wanted peace, the IRA wrote him off as a traitor." He turned to the window, gazing again. "If Conon O'Reilly was involved in his father's death—in serious trouble like that—would he go back to Miss Broderick?"

Did he make it? Abigail had asked. Jonas leaned forward. "About that compassionate leave, sir?"

"It's been denied."

Jonas tapped O'Reilly's picture. "Would it be if it related to this man?"

"Does it, Willoughby?"

"It could. I would recognize him."

"Are you risking another promotion?"

Jonas smiled. "I won't qualify for one as long as I'm at Northwood. The base isn't big enough for too many captains."

"Perhaps a few days' leave but working directly under me. You won't risk your career going after this man?"

"Wasn't that part of your plan, sir, part of your Irish project for me to find out whether he's there or not?"

"Go cautiously, Willoughby. But don't rule anyone out. Whoever is protecting the young terrorist would have close Irish-Catholic connections."

"Not necessarily, sir. Religion may not enter in. It might be the least likely person, someone with a motive of his own."

"Or *her* own?" McInytre suggested.

Jonas attempted to steer his thoughts from Abigail. "Maybe someone living there had a relative shot by the British Army. Something like that. Something he saw. Some injustice that colored his view of the establishment. What happened to my fiancée certainly colored my views. But I am a naval officer, sir. First and foremost. I have absolute loyalty to the Queen."

"I'm glad." McIntyre's attention once more focused on the view from his window. Suddenly, he whirled his chair around to face Jonas. "How much do you really know about Miss Broderick?"

"She's been part of my memories for a lifetime."

"And, as you've already pointed out, Willoughby, she would never let anything happen to any of her children. If this Conon O'Reilly is in England, I would think he would go to her."

"That's what I have to find out, sir."

"Broderick—is she British?"

"Decidedly, through and through. You don't think the Admiral would have a foreigner living at the manor all these years?"

"The children have been foreigners," McIntyre pointed out.

"Agreed. But Abigail knows no creed or nationality where her children are concerned."

"Then she might hide O'Reilly if he sought her help."

Moments later a clerk entered the room. "I've brought the folder you requested, sir."

"Good. Give it to me."

McIntyre scanned it. When he looked up, he said, "Brief as it is, this is all we have for you. O'Reilly belongs to a group that calls themselves 'the real IRA.' These are men who refuse to lay down their arms for any Good Friday Agreement. They don't want peace; they want war. Conon was involved in the bombing in Omagh. Been on the run ever since." He closed the folder. "He got his just due. Lost his wife in Omagh, poor devil."

"So he married? What a mess he's made of his life."

"I'm going to clear a month's leave for you, Willoughby. I want you to go back to Stow-on-the-Woodland and find out if O'Reilly has put in an appearance." Shrewdly, he added, "Stow-on-the-Woodland is a highly unlikely place to harbor a terrorist. But if you find him, Willoughby?"

"I'll bring him in, sir."

"It might cost you Broderick's friendship."

"She knows my loyalties."

"The question is, do you know hers?"

Eleven

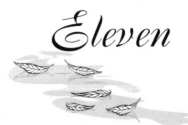

As she ran for the boarding gate at Kennedy International, Sydney was hemmed in by the vast crowd going nowhere, going everywhere. She prayed for a miracle to be on time—and for a second miracle to calm her lingering fears about flying out over Long Island, on the same route that her parents had taken.

Muffled bedlam echoed around her as she handed her passport to the attendant at the VIP counter. The agent's brow puckered. "There seems to be a mix-up. All we have left is an aisle seat."

"My window seat was guaranteed when I made my reservation."

The man behind her leaned forward. "Here, I don't mind an aisle seat. Why don't we switch?"

"You won't mind?" Sydney asked, whirling around to face the man and then exclaiming, "Jeff!"

Jeff VanBurien grinned. "One and the same. My travel agent pulled strings. We thought you could do with a friend on board."

"Then I won't have to fly alone."

"And I fly in the company of a beautiful woman."

Another tiny scowl knit the agent's brow. "We're already boarding first class, so hurry—and have a wonderful flight."

"We will." Jeff scooped up his case and Sydney's carry-on and led the way. As they cleared security and walked down the long ramp, he said, "I'm here as your friend, Syd. I figured this might be your first long-distance flight. Right?"

"Since Mom and Dad? Yes."

He stooped as they entered the cabin, the light catching the amber in his hair. "For months after we met, I studied everything about that crash—looking at the passenger list and wondering who those people were and why their lives were cut short."

"Why would you be allowed to do that?"

"My firm filed a lawsuit for one of the families."

Sydney glanced toward the pilot's cabin. "I still think it was pilot error," she whispered. "It must have been."

"No, the reports were accurate. The engine malfunctioned."

"I don't know whether to be nervous that you're on board talking like this or not."

"Just good therapy. It's bottled up inside of you. Let's get it out." He stowed her suitcase into a luggage hold. "Just consider me your guardian angel. I'll be sitting right beside you. If you need me, I'm only a hug away. Just say the word."

She fought off tears and gave an extra tug to her seat belt. Her knuckles turned chalk white as the jet rumbled full throttle down the runway and soared into the cloudless sky. Jeff's broad hand covered hers. "Open your eyes, sweetheart, and take a look."

She forced herself to peer through the smudged windows, down on the water sparkling in the fading sunlight. She remembered that other night. The long wait. The debris floating on top of the waves. The makeshift memorial service on the edge of the Sound days later. Suddenly that choppy sea lost its grip on her, for in remembering, the warmth of faces dear to her came back. She pictured her parents holding hands on takeoff, her dad grinning reassuringly. She knew that if they were capable of knowing, they would wish her well, loved her dearly. They'd left her a legacy of love more precious than the possessions that were hers now.

Gently, Jeff turned her face toward him. "You're okay?"

She met his gaze. "Okay."

Tweaking his mustache, he murmured, "About that problem you gave me—I've been wading knee-deep in law books on probate and British law. But your worries cost me extra money."

"How so?"

"I packed half my library in another suitcase."

Surely he joked, but she said, "Charge it to Barrington."

His grin broadened. "Already did. Have you heard any more from that bamboozler in England?"

"Edmund Gallagher? I called to confirm my arrival time and talked to another gentleman." She used the term lightly. "He was probably another member of Gallagher's firm."

"So what are your plans when we touch down at Heathrow?"

"I have a rental car waiting. Then straight to the Ritz."

"You're going in style. My brother's meeting me. We could give you a lift to your hotel and to the Cotswolds the next day."

"I need my own transportation. I scheduled time at the shipyard, but I should be in the Cotswolds by the weekend."

An hour into the journey—safely beyond the place where her parents' jet spiraled into the ocean—Sydney leaned her cushioned seat back as far as it would go and allowed Jeff to tuck her blanket around her. She caught his hand and pressed it to her cheek. "Thanks, Jeff. You're a rock."

He kissed her ear. "I wish I could be more."

Fifteen miles from Stow-on-the-Woodland, wisteria climbed the face of a row of honey-colored cottages with dormer windows and brass latches on their doors. Once domestic homes, they had been converted into business establishments—a pub, a tearoom, a small postal depot, and a solicitor's office. A gold-lettered sign creaked on its hinge above the cottage on the corner: *Edmund Gallagher, Solicitor.*

Inside, two volatile men burned the midnight oil in another heated argument about the problems at Broadshire

114

Manor. As the shouting grew louder, Edmund shuttered the windows and then stomped back to his father's old desk. His now.

From behind thick-rimmed glasses, he fixed his scornful gaze on Marshall Wallis. "Sit down, Marshall. I think we should deal with this like gentlemen."

Wallis kept pacing, his hands jammed into his pockets. "We have problems if you persist in laying claim to Broadshire Manor. Don't you understand that?"

"You have problems, my dear doctor. I'm only here two days a week—on loan from my law firm in London."

Edmund favored his lavish office in downtown London, but this country office was amply equipped with upscale furnishings that belied the ancient exterior of the building. Mentally he found himself despising Marshall for his simple tastes in life, his bent toward honesty. Edmund could take him down legally for betraying patient confidentiality; he preferred using him.

"My dear Marshall, it was your professional opinion that Abigail Broderick was on her deathbed."

"She's still running on borrowed time."

Edmund remained practical. "Then all we have to do is settle matters with the American. I'm certain I convinced her in our last phone conversation that I could handle the paperwork for her. Don't look so alarmed, Doctor. I'll make certain she receives a substantial settlement, and that will be it."

Marshall glanced at his watch. "Given the time difference between our two countries, Miss Barrington is already in flight. Her plane should reach Heathrow later this morning."

Edmund exploded. "How do you know that?"

Marshall dropped into the chair. "I answered your phone the other day while waiting for you."

"And you didn't tell me?"

"It must have slipped my mind, Edmund."

"That fool woman. I saw no need for her coming over here."

"Apparently, she did."

"We must keep her away from Broadshire Manor."

"How? Should I quarantine the place? What's happened to you, Edmund? You used to be a reasonable man."

"When I took over my father's office, all I found were promissory notes. Clients who never paid their bills. My father could have been a rich man. I intend to be one."

"Surely something good came out of your father's life."

"Yes. I learned that Abigail Broderick is the owner of Broadshire Manor. And that fit right in with my plans."

"Poor Abigail. She trusted you with her legal matters."

"She trusted my father more."

Edmund considered for a moment, tapping his thumbs together. "Perhaps the safest plan is to let Miss Barrington think that Abigail is buried in St. Michael's churchyard. We can change one of the markers. That way Miss Barrington won't be nosing around."

"You have a major problem. Abigail is not dead."

"I'm depending on you."

"You are crazy, Edmund. I'm doing my best to keep her alive. And I've lived long enough to regret our chance encounter in the London Club six months ago."

"So you keep telling me, but you're the one who broke into Lady Willoughby's sealed medical file. And you were more than anxious to share the secret that only your father knew about."

"Those were the worst forty minutes of my life. You pushing a wine glass toward me. Begging me to tell you more."

"As I recall, you enjoyed telling me everything."

"I was drunk," Marshall said. "Dead drunk."

"You never could handle wine, but you handed me what I needed to know." And what a triumph it had been. He could still hear himself saying, *So Jonas is not Lady Willoughby's son? Marshall, you have just given me the key to Broadshire Manor. I will turn that property into a resort and open up Stow-on-the-Woodland to tourism. It will be just a beginning.*

And poor Marshall, helpless as he had been that night, was right. Edmund had been scheming the way he did when they were boys. Intimidating his classmates. Bullying the younger boys. Conniving to win his way to the top. But Marshall had been guilty of sharing his father's private medical records.

"You will go on helping me, Marshall. How long do you think you would last at the health center if people knew you couldn't be trusted with their medical confidences?"

"I'll resign."

"And where would you go? Back to London? I will ruin any attempt you make to practice medicine in the city. Admiral Willoughby is still well known there. How far do you think you could go once it was known that you had ruined the reputation of the Admiral and his family?"

"Lady Willoughby is dead. Let it rest, Edmund."

"How can I? The property belonged to Lady Willoughby's family for generations, so what persuaded her to bypass husband and son and leave it to someone outside the family? Some secret? Some problem? Something more than Lady Willoughby's inability to bear a child? . . . The Admiral was a lady's man, wasn't he?"

Marshall sprang from his chair and started for the door.

"I'm not finished, my friend. Don't rush off."

Marshall paced again. "Edmund, the people in Stow-on-the-Woodland still revere the Admiral as an officer and a gentleman."

"Gentlemen sometimes make mistakes. It must have been a serious one to force Lady Willoughby to write Jonas and the Admiral out of her will." He drummed his fingers on one of his law books. "Lady Willoughby didn't live long enough to correct her error, but Abigail wants to hand over the property to a total stranger. And I must stop her. I want that property."

Tonight Marshall's ordinary features burned with resentment. "Jonas Willoughby is the rightful owner to Broadshire Manor."

"Except for this legal document, Marshall. It's called a will. Jonas is not in Abigail's will, but he was never interested in living in the Cotswolds. . . . Pacing like that, Doctor, is not good for your health. You'll end up ill like Miss Broderick."

Marshall slouched back into the chair. "Blast you, Edmund."

"Did you know she called me in London days before her heart attack?"

"We never discussed her private business."

"Not even about the children?"

"Of course, we discuss the children. I'm their doctor."

"Abigail wanted to drive into my London office to reverse her will. As she told me, she wanted Jonas to have what is rightfully his." He swiveled his chair. "I suggested waiting until I could make an appointment for her in the village. Fortunately for me, her heart prevented her from keeping that appointment. Jonas will be dumbfounded by the conditions of the will, but he won't argue with it. He's too much of a gentleman." Edmund tapped the desk. "Not too long ago, I offered to buy the place from Miss Broderick while Jonas was away at sea."

"At rock-bottom price?"

"At that time, I thought she was having financial difficulty running the manor. She should have found any offer satisfactory. The Admiral was in no condition to sign his funds over to her, and then, somehow she received funds from a Swiss account." The drumming intensified. "After that she told me the manor was not for sale. Ever. That she did have funds to cover the necessary repairs. But that was before you told me about Lady Willoughby's past. Perhaps your Miss Broderick held something over Lady Willoughby's head."

"Abigail's not that kind of woman."

"You are a physician, Marshall. Don't you know that we all have a dark side—even your precious Miss Broderick? I'd be fair about it. I would arrange everything—have the Admiral declared incompetent, if need be, and pension off the staff. Social Services can deal with the children. You'll thank me in time, Marshall. Developing Stow-on-the-Woodland will increase your practice at the health center."

"What makes you think Jonas Willoughby will let you take control? Have you forgotten his unwavering loyalty to Miss Broderick and the Admiral?"

Edmund adjusted his spectacles. "Jonas will do anything to protect his father's reputation—even if Abigail must lose the manor over it. And I will be there with a check already written out. She'll grab at it."

Marshall rubbed the back of his neck. "You will destroy Jonas in the process. Ruin his Navy career. Abigail will give you the property before she would let that happen."

"Jonas's Navy career is of no concern to me. Nor is preserving the Admiral's unblemished reputation. Building Stow-on-the-Woodland into a bustling tourist attraction is. And I need Broadshire Manor to accomplish that."

Marshall left the firm by the side door, unchained his bicycle, and started home by light of the stars and the headlamp on the cycle. Of all the villagers, Abigail brought him particular joy beyond his work at the health clinic. He admired her sacrifice, her mothering, mentoring ways with children. Telling her that she had to slow down for the sake of her heart had been received with the same philosophical approach that she tendered to any major decision. She would rest when she settled the plight of the children under her care.

As he rode the path along the Windrush, his heart thumped in beat with the pumping. A cramp started in the calf of his leg. He abandoned the ride to work the cramp from his leg and then pushed his cycle the last kilometer of the way.

At the crest of the hill, Stow-on-the-Woodland lay before him, asleep except for a light in Jonas Willoughby's cottage. So Jonas was back for the weekend? Beyond the cottage stood the manor, bleak in the darkness with only a tiny night-light in Abigail's bedroom window. He should go to her—see whether she had need of him. But what else could he do? Abigail's recovery lay in her own determination, not in the medicines he prescribed.

Marshall had only a stone's throw to go to reach the safety of his own bed, the warmth of his wife beside him. Instead he lowered his cycle to the ground, sat down on the small mound, and put his head in his hands. He never intended to betray a friend. In the quiet communing with his own soul, he had no choice but to go back in time to when he was still a lad. To when he most admired Lady Willoughby.

May, 1969. Marshall Wallis had just turned seven when he first saw Lady Willoughby at the village church, in a sanctuary packed to overflowing with Londoners. He swung his bare legs in the church pew, his hymnbook upside down as he watched her. She sat across the aisle from him, her widebrimmed spring hat shading her face. Her small son huddled beside her. Lady Willoughby sang in a voice high and crystal clear like the Windrush. In the middle of the hymn, she turned and smiled at him, her eyes as blue as the sky, her skin golden like the Cotswold Hills.

Later, as the service ended, she patted his head. "I'm Lady Willoughby. What is your name?"

"Marshall Wallis," he stammered.

"The doctor's son! Your father is a fine gentleman. Dr. Wallis has tended the Admiral for years. And now he's my doctor."

"Are you sick?"

"Sometimes." She smiled down at her son. "And your father takes care of Jonas too."

"Was Jonas one of my father's babies?"

She shook her head, amused. "Jonas was born in the north country. Now that you've met us, do come the next time your father calls at the Broadshire Manor."

As they walked down the aisle of St. Michael's, her frilly pink dress swished and the silk shawl around her shoulders fanned out light and breezy. Lady Willoughby smelled sweetly like the flowers on the altar; his mother smelled like cookies and greasy lamb. And there as a boy for the first time in his life, he knew that women were different, special, and he knew when he grew up that he would want to marry someone like Lady Willoughby.

Outside he stammered, "Lady Willoughby, do you have a bigger boy for me to play with when I come to see you?"

"Just Jonas. Will that matter? Yes, I see that it does. But we have horses, and Mrs. Quigley makes the best sweets in town."

They had reached the massive door of the church, and Marshall hurried past the ugly gargoyles that overshadowed St. Michael's. He looked back and saw Lady Willoughby still standing on the top step, the clergyman bending down to talk to the child beside her. *Just Jonas. Just a little boy.*

But Marshall did like horses and sweets and the flowery smell of Lady Willoughby as she walked past him.

On his first visit to the manor, Lady Willoughby had taken him to the stables and introduced him to her horse, Lightning. The horse had nuzzled her hand, nibbling the sugar cubes. "No one else rides him but me, Marshall," she had said.

After that, he often saw her racing across the valley, up the hills, over the glens into the woodland. He was twelve the day she died. He was riding in the car beside his father on their way back from his father's medical rounds. "Oh, stop, Father. That's Lady Willoughby and Lightning. Look at them go."

Smiling, his father pulled to the side of the road and left his engine idling. They watched Lady Willoughby racing across the crest of the hill, ladylike and graceful. She turned to wave at them, and suddenly horse and rider stumbled and fell.

Marshall and his father were the first to reach her. The stallion lay neighing, helplessly trying to stand again. "We'll have to put him down," his father said.

Lady Willoughby lay crumpled beside her horse, her beautiful face twisted, the green hillside blotched with her blood. Marshall stood immobilized as his father knelt by her side and slipped his hand beneath her neck.

He shook his head. "Her neck is broken, son."

"You're not going to put her down, Dad?"

"Stay calm, Marshall. Be brave for Lady Willoughby."

Even as the crowd gathered, he turned away, bent over, and vomited. He was still retching when they put the horse down.

For three days his father said nothing about the accident. Then, the day before the funeral, he called Marshall to his side. "I am driving into Cheltenham to see the pathologist."

He put his hands on Marshall's shoulders. "Drive along with me, son. This has been a hard lesson for you, watching Lady Willoughby die. I think you want to know why your friend died."

"Lightning threw her."

"But the pathologist will tell us medically how she died."

His lips were so dry he wasn't certain he could get the words out. "The man who did the autopsy? We're going there?"

"You don't have to go, son. You know that."

He had gone but not into the room with the pathologist. He stood near the open door watching his father flip through a file folder. "She was a beautiful woman," his father said.

"Not when I saw her, Wallis."

Five minutes later, his father thumped the chart and said, "This can't be true. Lady Willoughby has a son."

"Did you deliver the boy?"

122

His father sounded ruffled. "No, she was in the north country. Went there with a staff member."

"I'm telling you, Wallis, I have examined her and—"

"Hush. My son will overhear you."

The pathologist lowered his voice, but Marshall heard him say, "I'm sorry about the boy, Wallis, but let me remind you I know Lady Willoughby's body better than anyone now. I'm telling you, it would have been impossible for her to bear a child."

"But she has a son—a young lad away at Gordonstoun. He's coming home for the funeral. She definitely has a son."

The pathologist remained adamant. "But not a son from her own womb."

Twelve

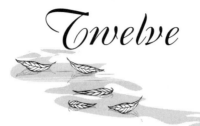

A night shadow fell across the silver on Marshall's bicycle. Before he could move, an iron grip dug into his shoulder. He tried to wrench free but could only turn his head and look up. "Jonas, what are you doing here?"

The grip loosened. "Dr. Wallis! I was about to ask you the same thing. Is everything okay with you? With your wife?"

"It won't be if I don't get home."

He dropped down beside Marshall. "When I saw someone riding along the Windrush at this hour, it didn't sit right with me."

"You thought I was the intruder? He's gone by now."

"Not so. He was injured. I think someone is harboring him here in the village. A wounded man might seek you out, Doctor."

"What about you, Jonas? Why did you leave town that night?"

"Are you wondering whether the stranger rode out of town with me?" There was amusement in Jonas's voice. "I'm hardly the man to protect an Irish rebel. No, I left town alone. Abigail begged me to go back to Northwood for my own protection."

"Why would she do that?"

Jonas drew his feet across the wet dew and encircled his knees. "She said she didn't want me involved in any ruckus in town, but I think she knows more about what happened that night than either one of us. I wish I could believe that she really wanted to protect me by sending me away."

"She'd do anything to save your career and reputation."

They fell silent, listening to the ripple of the Windrush. Marshall had not fully understood as a boy, but he had guessed from the expression on his father's face that shame stalked the Admiral and his family. Now, sitting on the crest of the hill beside the Admiral's son, it came back fresh and searing: *Lady Willoughby had not brought Jonas into the world.*

"Doctor," Jonas said, "how is Abigail doing? Really? She seemed stronger this morning when I had tea by her bedside."

"Don't get your hopes too high, Jonas. Her body is worn out, battened down with a soggy heart. I'm surprised she's clung to life so long. She might have had a better chance if we had hospitalized her in the beginning, but she refused to go to Cheltenham or London and leave Sir James and the children."

"No one is blaming you, Doctor."

"She wouldn't even accept health visitors around the clock. As weak as she was, she told me Mrs. Quigley would browbeat any intruder. She seems to feel safe in Mrs. Quigley's care."

"They've been great friends for years."

The doctor heaved a sigh. "I cautioned her to slow down and give her heart a rest, but I knew she would never do so. Now it doesn't look good. What's going to become of the place when—"

Jonas's features were mere shadows in the darkness. "When I first came home, I consulted Edmund Gallagher about the legality of selling the property while Dad and Abigail were still alive. Now I have doubts about letting the place go. They have the right to live out their lives here. Abigail loves the Cotswolds. She will go nowhere else. This is her little part of England."

"Edmund won't like being crossed."

"Selling is not his decision. He's going to have to tell his buyer that the manor isn't for sale." His voice grew husky.

"When I retire from the Navy, I might want to come back for good."

Marshall flattened his palm on the wet grass. "Your father and Abigail will both be dead by then. Maybe you should think of marrying and moving away."

"You know I thought about marrying. Louise and I planned to live in the manor. It will be lonely without her, but I'm going to like rambling around in that old house. It's filled with good memories. Mother. Louise. Abigail and her children. Think about it, Marshall. When Dad dies, I'll be lord of the manor. Sounds strange, doesn't it?"

Sounds complicated, Marshall thought.

With a quick spring, Jonas pushed to a standing position. "Can you spare the time to do some trout fishing tomorrow?"

"I'd like that, Jonas."

"I'll have Gregor with me. He's become my tagalong."

"Good lad, that one. He'll be lost when you go back to sea."

"I don't dare think about it." He brushed his hands. "Now that I know that it's you up here at 3:00 in the morning, I'll head back and get some sleep. Gregor tends to appear at my door at the crack of dawn."

"Take care, Jonas, and God bless."

"What?"

"I said 'God bless you.'"

He felt Jonas's eyes boring down on him. "My mother used to say that when I was a small boy and she tucked me in."

"Lady Willoughby used to say it to me too when I made house calls at the manor with my father. She was a good woman, Jonas. A beautiful woman."

"I was only eight when Mother died."

"I was twelve. In many ways, Abigail reminds me of her."

"How so?"

"That inner strength. Her devotion to the Admiral and you. Abigail has that same womanly grace that I admired in

Lady Willoughby." *Her own measure of beauty,* Marshall thought. *A face sculpted by the hands of the gods.*

"That's good of you to say. Abigail's the one who forced me to go on riding horses after Mother's accident. I'll always be grateful to her. She's always been there for me." He reached out and gripped Marshall's hand. "Come on. On your feet, man. Go home and get some rest. Whatever is bothering you should look better in the morning. Good night."

"Good night, Jonas."

The clammy feeling came back as Jonas strolled off. A man went fishing with his friends, not with a man he was betraying.

Dawn held another dread. Before the sun bathed the Cotswold Hills in golden splendor, Miss Barrington's plane would touch down at Heathrow—a rich young woman coming here to claim her inheritance from a woman who so far refused to die.

Marshall had solved nothing by remembering the past, nothing by sitting on the hillside, yet his resolve stood firm. He would protect his friends at the manor whatever it cost him. Today he would tell his wife that his job was at stake. Yet he sensed only guilt at the thought of sharing Lady Willoughby's secret with another human being.

Jeff VanBurien leaned through the open window of the rental car and kissed Sydney on the cheek. "Are you certain you don't want us to follow you into London?"

"Jeff, I'll be okay. I've been here many times."

"Drive carefully."

"I won't go a kilometer over the limit. How's that?"

"Do you have a map marked out for the trip to the Tyne?"

"Right in my briefcase. And I have the trip mapped out to Stow-on-the-Woodland. You're beginning to sound like Randolph."

"And that's not good." He stepped back and stood beside his half-brother, Chandler Reynolds. Sydney turned the key in the ignition and smiled at them both. "Chan, I'm sorry I missed your wife."

"Couldn't be helped. Jillian is in Rome for a fortnight. I hope she'll be back before you leave."

"Does she always holiday alone?"

A teasing good humor settled in Chandler's eyes. "This is a business trip. She's tracking another stolen masterpiece. Lot of theft of the art masters in Italy. But you mentioned Stow-on-the-Woodland. Do you have friends there, Sydney?"

"No, but I have property. I just inherited some land when a friend died."

Chandler frowned. "It's not a big village."

"The solicitor called my place Broadshire Manor."

Chandler's answer seemed to stick in his throat. Jeff nudged him. "Something wrong, fella?"

"My wife talked about that place on the phone last evening."

"Small world," Jeff told him.

"I have to run," Sydney said. "You have my number, Jeff. I'm counting on your help."

"I can hardly forget the name Sheepfold. I'll leave any messages for you there. And you have Chan's number in London?"

She patted the briefcase beside her. "I have it." She blew Jeff a kiss. "Thanks for traveling with me. I mean it."

"My pleasure. Now remember. Don't sign anything. Not until you discuss it with me."

"Agreed. That's what I'm paying you for."

She backed out of the rental lot and drove off with a quick wave. As her car turned out of sight, Jeff faced his brother. "Chan, are you going to wipe that frown off your face or are you going to tell me what's wrong? I thought you'd like Sydney."

"I do, and I'm not sure anything's wrong, but it seems unlikely that there are two Broadshire Manors in that village."

"And that bothers you?"

"What bothers me is my wife having dinner in Rome with her old boyfriend, Santos Garibaldi."

"Should I step aside and let you fly down there?"

"Jillian wouldn't thank me for that. She's in Rome on an art fraud case. But, Jeff, you didn't tell me you were traveling over here with a beautiful woman. Is it serious with this Sydney Barrington? And not a hint of it in our phone calls?"

"I'm not in her class, Chan."

"But you'd like to be?"

"What man wouldn't?"

Chandler grinned as he brushed his hand through his red-brown hair. "Me for one. I found myself when I found Jillian."

"So what about her old boyfriend?"

"Santos Garibaldi? He contacted Jillian the minute he heard she was in Rome. He lives there. Told her he needed her help."

"That's a new line."

"Jillian believed him the minute he told her he was concerned about art treasures disappearing in Stow-on-the-Woodland. Seems Santos spent part of his boyhood growing up there. As a thank-you, his father sculpted a fountain in front of Broadshire Manor. They apparently have a number of valuable paintings inside the manor."

"Then it's no small cottage Sydney's inherited?"

"Right. And according to Jillian, this Miss Broderick is ill but not dead. There's no way Sydney can inherit the place, not when it belongs to a retired Admiral in the Royal Navy who is still very much alive."

Jeff smoothed his mustache with his thumb and forefinger. "I get the feeling we're not talking about the same place."

"I think we are."

"That doesn't make sense. The lawyer who contacted Sydney said Abigail Broderick *was* dead. He wanted to settle everything by long distance. That didn't sit well with Syd. Nor with me when she told me about it. But I'm positive there was no mention of any valuable paintings."

"The lawyer wouldn't mention them if he wanted them for himself. And if Abigail Broderick had died, I'm sure Santos would have mentioned it to Jillian. He's apparently quite fond of the old girl."

"Could we drive out there tomorrow and nose around, Chan?"

"Sure. It's only an hour and half from London. We'll make it part of our holiday."

"What's in it for Santos besides picking up a marble statue and taking it back to Rome? What is it? Another Trevi Fountain?"

Chandler laughed. "Santos appreciates art. What true Italian wouldn't? But he has it in his head that he has to protect the art at Broadshire Manor. According to Jillian, he's kept in touch with Miss Broderick over the years and knows that she's seriously ill. He's flying back from Rome when Jillian comes home."

He clicked his remote keyless entry. "Here we are."

They had reached Chan's van and stood on opposite sides, facing each other across the rooftop. *Brothers. The same bloodline. But people would take us for total strangers,* Jeff thought. He felt even more rail-thin looking at his brother's muscular body. London and marriage had been good for Chan; he had the look of a happy man.

"We'd better go," Chan said, ducking into the van. Jeff followed his lead and fastened his seat belt. "Do you think Sydney is all right traveling alone, Jeff?"

"She's an independent lady. She'll make it. But I promised her we'd be here for her."

"You're over here as her lawyer, aren't you?"

He reached out and squeezed Chandler's shoulder. "Helping Sydney is just an added bonus. Mostly, I came to spend a holiday with my kid brother."

"I've been looking forward to your visit for months, Jeff."

"I marked it on my calendar back in January."

Jeff heaved a happy sigh as their vehicle merged with the traffic. It would be all right. They stood on a solid foundation—two brothers seeking to know each other better.

Thirteen

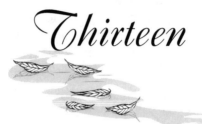

As she left the Jarrow Shipyard on Saturday, Sydney wore her windbreaker as a safeguard against the unpredictable English weather. After two days of inspecting the progress at the shipyard and climbing around the construction site in a hard hat and a borrowed khaki jumper, she felt satisfied that things were moving on schedule. With a wave to the weekend foreman, she left the plant and nosed her rental car toward the Cotswolds—to the land and children she had inherited.

With her company's reputation and that deeply ingrained Barrington confidence, she had no doubt she could win the carrier contract. But she wanted someone who had worked by her side to oversee that long-term project. Her architect Daron Emery knew the carrier blueprints best and had been in on the initial designs. The job would be safe in Daron's hands. With that firmly settled in her mind, she was able to put the shipyard behind her and turn her thoughts completely to the journey ahead.

An hour later she pulled off the motorway and placed a call to Edmund Gallagher's Cotswold office. For the third time since arriving in England, she was forced to leave a message on his answering machine. Was he just out of the office or had he changed his mind about their appointment at noon today?

Back in the car, Sydney decided to drive straight through to Stow-on-the-Woodland. She had no intention of meeting Gallagher in the blind or having him shove papers across the desk for her to sign for a property sight unseen. She'd drive by Broadshire Manor for a glimpse and then journey back to Bourton-on-the-Water where she was staying. That meant little more than a thirty-mile delay in her arrival time at the bed-and-breakfast. Still, she had an uncanny feeling that Jeff VanBurien would frown at this decision.

Leaving the motorway, she drove the narrow two-lane road, delighting in the scent of country air and the fragile tapestry of the hills in burnished gold. She would have known without the road signs that she had entered the Cotswolds. The evidence surrounded her: limestone slopes alive with wildflowers and grazing cattle, gardens overgrown with primrose climbers, thatched cottages and aristocratic estates that seemed to dominate each village. The road climbed and dipped into more secluded valleys, through wooded ravines, and along the banks of the river where alders and cottonwoods grew. Village after village, evoking a time gone by.

In Bourton-on-the-Water, she eased along High Street and spotted Gallagher's office. It was closed. Fifteen miles later, she came to Stow-on-the-Woodland and parked the car by the River Windrush. As she emerged from the car, the unspoiled countryside snatched her breath away. She had stepped into another time, yet it was timeless. Everything familiar stood still; everything new had been set in motion. A sweeping calm engulfed her as though some fragment of her life was coming together, some part of her future taking shape. The hills and meadows were flecked with an unending stretch of buttercups. On both sides of the river lay clusters of honey-buffed homes as ancient as her forefathers.

The past became a charming present. High-gabled buildings with dates carved into their chipped walls. Cozy shops along the narrow streets with bright metal shingles announcing their wares. A church with a fifteenth-century spire and lean, leafy trees lining the footpath to it. Seeing the high, rolling wolds, she knew she must find a horse and saddle to rent so she could explore those golden-green slopes where land and horizon met.

But there was no need to ask for directions to Abigail Broderick's place. A magnificent country home dominated the scene. If that was indeed Broadshire Manor, Sydney had come into a sizable possession that stirred more questions and concern than when she first heard about a piece of land and six children. She imagined that history had placed it there with its commanding view of the valley and that the fortunes and failures of this village were linked with the family who owned it. Was Abigail Broderick a member of an aristocratic family? Gallagher had painted her as an ordinary country woman.

Sydney retraced her steps and sat down near the water's edge, close to the village green. The crystal-clear Windrush that had been here forever, rippled along through the center of town. The marvelous gurgling, bubbling sound of water running free. It splashed over the rocks and squeezed past the rush-tangled banks as it meandered on its way. It seemed to Sydney she had been here before, as though she had come home. She leaned down and let the river wash over her hand. Again, that simple act felt familiar.

As she drew her hand from the Windrush, a little girl as pale as the curtains in the storefront windows ran dangerously close to the water's edge, a young boy in angry pursuit. "Keeley, we must go home!" he shouted after her.

The girl stumbled to an abrupt halt in front of Sydney. Their eyes held over the grassy bank that separated them.

"Hello," Sydney said.

The child remained mute, her bright red curls falling softly around her face. As they sized each other up, shyness showed through those doelike eyes. She jerked free from the boy's grasp and ran again, this time in dizzying circles around Sydney.

Sydney understood the child's bid for freedom, the shyness. She reached out her hand to the girl—reached out her

134

hand to the child in herself. "Come. Sit with me here on the bank of the river."

Without a word, the child flopped down beside Sydney and leaned against her, trembling. Sydney drew the child closer.

Hesitating, not certain what to do with a stranger looking on, the boy said, "She's Keeley. I've come to take her home."

"Are you her brother?" They didn't look alike. His brilliant eyes were dark, his skin sun-brown.

"No. She lives with me up there."

He pointed back toward the country house at the crest of the hill. "That's a big house," Sydney said.

"It belongs to the Admiral."

Not to Abigail Broderick? Or had Edmund Gallagher already sold the land to some retired admiral and his family? But the children were still there. Still safe. The Admiral? She felt as enlightened as the peacock butterfly spreading its wings on the bush beside her. The boy reached out to rob it of its freedom.

"Don't do that," she commanded.

He pulled back, his shiny eyes staring hard at her. "I would not hurt it. I just wanted to feel it wiggling in my hand."

Her attention drew back to the manor. The property seemed to stretch on forever: a piece of land of sizable dimensions and six children. The oldest child was around nine, Gallagher had told her. This boy could easily be nine.

"Do you always come down here alone?" she asked.

"I have to. Keeley keeps running away."

"Perhaps she's unhappy."

"She's Irish."

The boy's thought process amused her. "Maybe I should walk up to the house with you," she offered.

"You coming for dinner? Mrs. Quigley don't like strangers uninvited."

His grammar was atrocious, but the English he knew had a decided British clip. Edmund Gallagher had said, "A Mrs. Quigley is watching over them."

A woman who didn't like uninvited guests.

"I should eat before I go up there." She glanced around at the shops and wondered where in this little hamlet she might find a hearty meal.

"Jonas goes to Chutman's Pub." His stubby finger indicated the quaint store on the corner.

Jonas? Another name, but apparently he had the boy's absolute respect and loyalty. His lustrous eyes glowed. "Or you can go to Veronica's Tea Shoppe." This time he pointed to a shop with a pink shingle. "Jonas buys me sweets there sometimes."

"Candy bars?"

He frowned, puzzled. "Chocolates. Mostly after I help him pull weeds or tend the sheep."

A hired hand for sure then, she thought. But a man well loved by this boy. "Why don't we go up to the house first?" she suggested. "I'll come back for supper later. I'd better know your name so I'll know who I'm following."

"I'm Gregor."

"And I'm Sydney."

He flashed a warm, friendly grin. "Come on."

She took Keeley's hand and felt the warmth of the child's in her own. Gregor ran ahead of them, doing leapfrogs and handstands and picking up pebbles from the ground. Still he made good mileage until he reached the twisted footpath that climbed toward the manor. He stopped and looked back. "You coming?"

"We're coming."

"We go through the woodland."

"Okay."

It was an easy climb. As Gregor rushed ahead, she thought, *There's an old beech tree just around that first corner where a clump of azaleas used to grow.* But it turned out to be a vine of musk orchids growing there. Her lips went dry. But somewhere. Somewhere back in time—

As they neared the manor, he let out a whoop. "Jonas is home!"

He was off running, in a straight line this time. Sydney set her pace to Keeley's, speaking of the beauty around them, of the shimmering Windrush behind them. They paused to touch a flower. Keeley felt the petals but said nothing. Perhaps she knew no English at all.

As they approached, the manor seemed even more imposing, the property immense and hedged in by a quaint dry-stone wall. It was a two-story structure, three if you counted the dormer windows on the upper level with its limited dwelling quarters. On a breezy day, it would take the brunt of the wind, its windows rattling and its eaves bending.

A flowering vine with ruby-red fronds climbed the face of the building, close to where another wing had been added. Off to the side of the house, Sydney could see the edge of the stables and a high water tower. A thatched cottage stood on the far corner, a car parked beside it.

But most intriguing was the marvelous fountain in front— a boy and girl in marble spewing a steady flow of water that turned to ribbons of color as the sun reflected through it. In the back of her mind, Sydney felt certain she had seen the statue before—as though she had actually heard the water cascading over the bare feet of the children a long time ago.

Her thoughts raced. Inherit this immense acreage and she would have to hire a large domestic staff and gardeners and someone to maintain the stables and plow the land—a more formidable task than being CEO at Barrington. As much as she disliked Edmund Gallagher, his plan could well be the better choice. She could parcel out the land to developers as he wanted to do. Or would pride force her to take it on as another opportunity to prove to Randolph Iverson that she could handle anything? Or would this become Sydney's folly—only a driving distance from the shipyard still known as Aaron's faux pas?

Gregor shoved open the gate and bounded to the gardener.

Sydney caught the gate with the palm of her hand as it swung back and noticed the family crest embedded in it. *Broadshire Manor: The Willoughbys.* On the other side of the drystone wall, the gardener was pruning the roses. She was struck by the strength of his broad shoulders, his sun-tanned skin. He yanked off his sun shades, further revealing his handsome, unsmiling face. But the second Gregor flung himself at the man, he tossed his spade in the wheelbarrow and gathered the boy to his side. He glanced over at Sydney and Keeley and nodded brusquely; there was no warm welcome for Keeley, only question marks in his frosty blue gaze.

"When'd you come, Jonas?"

"Two hours ago," he said. "You'd best take your guests inside and then get back and help me. Later we can bring the sheep in for Boris."

The boy raced back to Sydney, grinning. "I'm going to help Jonas. He just got home."

"I see that," she said. "Was he off buying garden supplies?"

"Boris does the shopping. Jonas was at Northwood."

Sydney felt the gardener's eyes still on her as she walked up the steps with Keeley dogging her heels and Gregor bounding up ahead of them. Twelve steps. She counted them. Twelve steps closer to possessing this land. She thought of the gardener's frosty blue eyes meeting hers; perhaps she would keep him on to man the flower beds. She reached over Gregor's head for the knocker, but he swung the massive door open for her.

"So there you are, Gregor," said a gravelly voice. "I sent you to get Keeley, not go on a picnic that took all morning."

"Keeley didn't want to come, Mrs. Quigley." He pointed his thumb backwards. "This lady helped me."

At the sight of the woman fanning herself with a makeshift apron, Keeley pressed against Sydney. "I thought Gregor needed help," Sydney apologized.

Mrs. Quigley was a tall, buxom woman. Wrinkled ridges cut deep into her face. The top button of her housedress lay open, revealing the sagging skin folds at her neck. Her eyes were stern, a faded green, but alert, not missing a thing as her ample body blocked the doorway. She was obviously a country woman, a member of the staff, yet overpowering with her grim expression.

But she gave Gregor's head an affectionate pat. "Go on with you. And take Keeley. I want you both washed up and back in the kitchen right away."

"Can I take the Admiral's tray up to him?"

"Not today, Gregor. Lucas came for it."

He glanced up at Sydney, his thumb pointing back at her again. "What about her? She's hungry."

"No, I only walked the children up here," explained Sydney. "Actually, I was looking for Broadshire Manor when I came to town."

"You found it. But you already know that. I saw you reading the family crest on the gate," Mrs. Quigley said accusingly.

"Yes: *The Willoughbys.* Somehow that wasn't what I expected."

"What were you expecting?"

"Abigail Broderick's name. Has the place already been sold?"

A shadow darkened Mrs. Quigley's face. "You're the American woman looking to take over the land?"

Sydney blushed at the accusation. "I'm Sydney Barrington."

"That's the name Dr. Wallis gave us. He was here today. Said you were to see the solicitor from Bourton-on-the-Water. We weren't expecting you to put in an appearance at the manor."

"I'm sorry. Everything was so beautiful, I just kept driving. I did call Mr. Gallagher, but he wasn't in."

"Odd, if he had an appointment, he'd be there. He thinks in terms of pounds and more pounds. He won't like it, you coming here first." But Mrs. Quigley flashed a whimsical smile as though she were delighted with Sydney's defiance.

"It's Saturday. Maybe he forgot our appointment."

"Dr. Wallis thought you were to see him in London."

She wondered who Dr. Wallis could be. "No, yesterday Mr. Gallagher definitely said his Cotswold office. I had an appointment to meet with him at noon today, but his office was closed."

"It sounds like he's avoiding you." It was Mrs. Quigley's turn to look puzzled. "Well, you are here now, so come on in." She shot a glance at Keeley as Gregor led her away. "Getting that one to move is worth a cup of tea. Getting her here without a tantrum is worth some stew and dumplings. That's what the rest of us are having. So come on in, Miss Barrington."

"I really should go back to the village tea shop."

"You think that's better than my cooking?"

"I really don't know. I haven't tried either one. I know this is an awkward time for me to put in my appearance. Truly, I'm sorry about Miss Broderick."

The cagey eyes narrowed, a tear brimming on the eyelash. "She spent too much time taking care of the children and the Admiral—and not that old heart of hers. Nobody could stop her."

As Sydney stepped inside, she said, "Mrs. Quigley, I thought the Admiral was—maybe the new owner?"

"New owner? This place has been in the Willoughby family for generations. And if I get my way, it will stay in this family. Actually, it belonged to Lady Willoughby, the Admiral's wife. I've been here for years, and there's never been a *For Sale* sign in front of Broadshire Manor. Never. I suppose you've been listening to that Edmund Gallagher and all his fancy ideas for expanding Stow-on-the-Woodland?"

The Admiral's property? Not Abigail Broderick's?

140

"I haven't met Mr. Gallagher yet. We've just talked on the phone. That's how I knew about the place—and the children. I think I don't really understand what's going on."

"Then you didn't fly over to buy the place?"

"Right now, I'm not sure why I'm here. I reserved a room at a bed-and-breakfast in Bourton-on-the-Water. I really should be getting back there."

"Wait. We need to talk first. Get some understanding between us. I'll make up a room for you. You can try phoning Mr. Gallagher again on Monday."

"Stay here?" She was thrilled at the prospect. "I'd have to get my car. I parked it down by the war memorial."

She snorted. "Left down there unattended it could become another war casualty. Coming here first won't sit well with Edmund, but I rather think Dr. Wallis will be pleased."

"I don't know Dr. Wallis."

"He runs the health center. Comes by here every day. But never mind. Boris will go for the car and bring it up. This is the last place Gallagher will be expecting to find you. You get a good night's rest—you'll need it before you talk to him."

The stranger did not go unnoticed by Jonas. He had watched her coming up the footpath from the center of town. He liked her easy, unhurried stride, but who was she? Why was she here? Would she and her little girl interfere in his search for the wounded man? She seemed to be soaking up the beauty of the Cotswold Hills as she paused to cup a flower in her fingers and to pluck a tree leaf for the child.

The thick foliage had shaded her features as she approached, but as she stepped through the gate, their eyes met briefly, curiosity in her gaze. She had an elegance of her own—beauty and stature, poise and gracefulness. She was lovely to look at with her chestnut-brown hair drawn back from her oval face. Brilliant brown eyes shone beneath arched brows. She was fashionable even in the slacks and blue sweater she was wearing, a successful-looking woman. A woman with a little girl of her own.

So busy was he watching her that he snipped his finger with the pruning shears. He grabbed a rag from the wheel-barrow to stem the flow of blood, but as Gregor ran back to the stranger, she had looked at Jonas once more. Their gaze locked across the primroses. Her skin was soft. Her lips full. A hint of laughter at her mouth. In that split second, Jonas sensed something familiar about her—as though she had stepped from his past to brighten his life again.

He watched her until she reached the top step, and then he turned away, embarrassed. He tossed his tools in the wheelbarrow and broke off a rose in full bloom. A rose for Louise. A rose for the stranger.

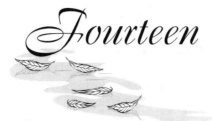

Fourteen

Jonas marked the restless night by tossing on his bunk until 2:00 in the morning with his thoughts on the possibility of Abigail harboring a fugitive. Niggling doubts crushed the image he held of her. She was in his memory, his mother's closest friend, the woman who had stepped in to comfort him when his mother died. Without her, his mailbox at Gordonstoun would have been empty, his holidays lonely. When he was older, she smothered her disappointment when he spent his holidays in the homes of his classmates and fellow officers. But even then, Abigail boasted about his career and defended him in front of the Admiral.

At Gordonstoun parental visits rarely exceeded three times a year. Jonas's Uncle Ian assumed this responsibility, not his father, and certainly not his mother's friend. She was too busy with her refugee children. Yet that day when he was only eight, he marched into the headmaster's office feeling small and insignificant in his gray jersey and corduroy trousers and found Abigail waiting for him.

"I have come to take you home, Jonas."

"I can't leave midterm."

The headmaster cleared his throat. "It is all right, Mr. Willoughby. You have permission to leave with Miss Broderick."

She had come to take him home for his mother's funeral, but even then she said, "Jonas, something has happened to Lady Willoughby and Lightning."

He thought it odd afterward that she had not said, "Something happened to your mother and her horse." But with Abigail, it was always *Lady Willoughby.*

As far back as he could remember, Abigail Broderick had surrounded herself with children, yet she always had time for him. She taught him respect for Margaret Thatcher and an unwavering admiration for the monarchy. She could trace the monarchy back for decades and considered the Queen a peer, so close were they in age. She spoke movingly of Princess Elizabeth making her first broadcast in 1940 to the children being evacuated from the London blitz. Jonas knew little of Abigail's past except that she had been engaged to a British commando, a man she had met on the beaches of Dunkirk. What had become of him, why she had never married, why she had never loved anyone else were matters that she kept to herself, making the mysteries that surrounded her even more intriguing.

But Abigail work against the British crown? Never. She would not betray the Queen. But would she risk hiding one of her children and consider it nonpolitical? He honestly did not know. One thing he knew with searing accuracy, however. Her prayers had followed him everywhere.

He had come back from Northwood yesterday with the full intention of taking Lucas into his confidence and enlisting his help. He felt a tie-in with any man who had served with the Royal Navy, a man loyal to his own father. Together they could search out Stow-on-the-Woodland cottage by cottage and comb through Broadshire Manor floor by floor, room by room. Corridor creeping at midnight, if need be. But did Jonas really expect to find Conon O'Reilly hiding out in some closet in the manor?

He piled his tools into the wheelbarrow and took them with him so he could get back to the primroses after breakfast. When he wheeled his equipment into the front yard, he spotted Gregor with the small redheaded girl in tow.

"Good morning, Gregor. Where are you going?"

"To the kitchen."

"Griselda has enough to do without children underfoot before breakfast. Where's the child's mother?"

"She didn't come with a mother. Just with her brother over there."

The girl turned her enormous eyes on the front door as a small boy propelled himself over the threshold and tumbled down the stone steps. Before he reached bottom, he was screaming.

Jonas scooped the boy up and covered the torn shin with his bare hand. Blood spurted through Jonas's fingers as he carried him up the steps and into the kitchen.

"Griselda, call Dr. Wallis. This child needs stitches."

She held a cooking pan in her hand, her eyes bulging. "The poor darling. What did you do to him, Jonas?"

"Do? I picked him up. Here, give me a towel. I've got to stop this bleeding."

She pushed him aside. "No need to bother Dr. Wallis. Let me look. I've been dealing with skinned shins for forty years."

"Who is he anyway?" Jonas asked.

"A guest at the manor."

"I saw a woman arrive yesterday—"

"A pretty woman never passed your notice." Immediately she murmured, "I'm sorry, Commander. It's just all the excitement lately. Cooking for the children. Caring for—"

"That woman should be down here taking care of her own children. I didn't realize she had two children. Has the whole family moved in? All this company is too upsetting for Abigail."

"Hush, or Miss Barrington will hear you," Griselda said as she cleaned the wound.

Miss Barrington? A name from his boyhood. He remembered the crush he had on the little girl from America. "That woman is Sydney Barrington? Did Abigail send for her?"

"No. Edmund Gallagher did. And she came alone."

"What about these children, Mrs. Quigley? Two little redheads. What are they doing here? Who are they?"

Gregor volunteered the answer. "Keeley and Danny O'Reilly."

"Jonas, they're Conon O'Reilly's children."

For a second Jonas stood immobilized. Speechless. Then anger rose and spilled over. "Conon O'Reilly's children? That's why you were so anxious to send me back to Northwood that night. You took a terrorist into this house? How dare you!"

"Calm yourself, Jonas. The children—"

"Where is he?"

"I don't know what you're talking about."

"Their father. Where is he?"

"He went away the night he left the children here."

Jonas saw Keeley's lip quiver, but he raged on. "Was that the night Abigail had her heart attack? I see by your silence that it was. Griselda, you can't keep the children of Conon O'Reilly in this house. I won't allow it."

"You don't expect me to throw them out, do you?"

"Where is Conon?"

"Gone."

"I intend to find him."

Griselda drew Danny into her lap and held him against her. "You're frightening this child."

"The accident frightened him. Have Boris take him to the doctor."

"No. Dr. Wallis comes later this morning. I'll have him check the leg then—once the American woman leaves."

Gregor murmured, "You said she's staying for the weekend."

"Oh, so I did. I invited her myself." Flustered, she reached out and patted Keeley's cheek. "It is all right, Keeley. No one will harm you. Gregor, get some sausage and scones for the children, will you?"

"When did you start serving sausage and scones for breakfast? You never served them to me."

"You didn't cut your leg, Jonas."

He was outraged. He looked at the injured child. Glared at the frightened sister. He felt sudden remorse as Keeley trembled uncontrollably. Above their heads, his gaze turned back to Griselda. "That child needs comfort too."

"She doesn't like sitting on my lap."

Gregor placed a bowl of sausage and scones on the table beside Griselda. "I think I'll go out, Mrs. Quigley."

"Why don't you take Keeley O'Reilly with you?" Jonas snapped. But Keeley darted past him, tears streaming down her face, and ran toward the east wing.

"Now see what you've done, Commander."

They endured a five-minute silence and then Jonas stomped to the stove and poured himself a boiling cup of tea. Without wincing, he swallowed and then turned his full rage on the woman who had nursed him through his childhood.

"I think you'd better pack up, Griselda, and leave—"

Sydney stretched contentedly on her bed, enjoying the old-fashioned luxury of her room with furnishings of English Oak dating back to the seventeenth century. The high headboard and four posters were carved with peacocks and floral buds. Above Sydney, the ceiling was designed with rosettes. *Her room.* She already thought of it as her own. She contemplated how she could rearrange the furniture and soften the colors with a pastel spread and curtains instead of the thick mauve drapes that had gathered dust into their folds. She would push her bed closer to the windows for the view and the fresh air of the country. And perhaps the gardener—and she flushed thinking of his handsome face— would cut her a fresh bouquet of flowers for her room.

Stop, she told herself. *You haven't seen Edmund Gallagher. The settling of a will takes time. The children. Yes, they would come first. They would have to take priority over remodeling.*

She was so engulfed in her own thoughts that she almost missed the clamor of voices outside and the sudden cry of a child in distress. Thoughts of Keeley sent her racing across the room. She leaned out the window and saw only the beauty of the landscape, the hills just as glorious as yesterday. The air was scented with intoxicating herbs.

As she watched, Gregor walked down the front steps with his hands jammed in the pockets of his short trousers, his head downcast. A picture of gloom on a sunny morning.

"Gregor, I heard someone crying. Is everyone all right?"

He shaded his eyes. "Danny fell down. Mrs. Quigley has him."

"Then he'll be all right?"

"Everybody is all right with Mrs. Quigley."

"Where's the gardener, Gregor?"

He shrugged. "The gardeners come on Monday."

"I mean the man who was pruning the roses yesterday. Jonas, you called him. I see his wheelbarrow out there."

"He's in the kitchen. He's mad at Mrs. Quigley."

And you're driving me mad, she thought smiling. "But I wanted him to pick me some wildflowers to take with me when I leave."

"Come down. I will help you pick them."

"I'll be there in fifteen minutes."

She bathed in an old tub with claw feet in a room with no lock on the door. After she dressed, she went back to her bedroom and found Keeley buried under the pillows. "What's wrong, sweetheart?"

"Danny fell down. And that man is mad at me."

The child had actually spoken. Sydney dropped onto the bed and encircled her. "Who's Danny?"

"My little brother. He's bleeding."

She panicked at the thought of any of the children hurt, unattended. "Honey, isn't Mrs. Quigley with him?"

"Yes, but I want you to come."

Keeley tugged at her hand and led her from the east wing, down the long corridor to the kitchen. They stopped short of the open door, Keeley shrinking against her. Sydney listened, shocked at a man's angry voice saying, "I think you'd better pack up, Griselda, and leave."

Sydney burst into the kitchen and stared at the rangy gardener lording it over Mrs. Quigley. "How dare you speak to Mrs. Quigley like that! Go back to your garden and take your anger out on the weeds and the rosebushes."

As he spun around to face Sydney, a lock of dark hair fell across his broad forehead. He swept it back, revealing a pinched frown wedged between his brows.

"You heard me. You can't talk to Mrs. Quigley that way. Just go back to your flowers and cool down."

For a moment, his frosty blue eyes seemed like dark circles. He looked as though he would turn his tongue-lashing on her. Instead the frost in his eyes melted and a bemused smile formed at the corners of his mouth. He took his teacup and deliberately poured the contents into the sink, then glancing briefly at Griselda, said, "We'll finish this later."

Jamming his hands into his pockets, he left the kitchen, but he was whistling.

"Who does he think he is?" Sydney asked when he was out of earshot. "A gardener talking to you like that?"

Mrs. Quigley's hand shook as she pulled Danny closer to her. "Everything will be fine, Danny," she said, but her voice trembled. "And I've got to get the rest of the children up and fed. And breakfast upstairs to—"

More gently Sydney said, "What right did he have to talk to you that way?"

"He has every right, Miss Barrington. He is the lord of the manor—at least he will be someday."

"Lord of the manor? The owner? He's—he's not the gardener?"

"No, he is Jonas Willoughby—the Admiral's son."

The admiral that Gregor had mentioned yesterday.

"But what about Miss Broderick? Oh, never mind—"

She had blown it. If she was up against an Admiral and his son, she felt certain the carrier bid would slip through her fingers.

"I guess I just don't understand what's going on."

"None of us do. Right now, with the Admiral ill, Jonas isn't himself. He has too much responsibility. On top of that he's stationed at Northwood."

"That Navy base near London?"

"Yes."

"Jonas is a serving officer in Her Majesty's Royal Navy. A Navy pilot really, but stuck on land now. I know the poor boy hates it. He had to give up so much when he found out about the Admiral and Abigail."

Sydney patted Griselda's shoulder. "It's all right. I'll apologize to Jonas. I'm so sorry for coming in the way I did. But he still doesn't have any right to talk to you that way."

"In a way he did. You see, he didn't know Danny and Keeley were staying here. He thought Keeley came with you."

"With me? He didn't know about these children?"

"Not about the O'Reilly children. He just came back from Northwood—just an hour or so before you saw him. He's been gone a couple of weeks. We wanted him to stay away from the excitement in Stow-on-the-Woodland."

"Excitement in this quiet little hamlet? It doesn't look like anything exciting ever happens here. It's so peaceful—"

Mrs. Quigley gave an indiscernible nod of her head toward Keeley. "I'll let Jonas explain things to you. You said you were going to apologize to him. I think that's best. Otherwise he will send these children away."

"That sounds like Edmund Gallagher."

"He's nothing like Mr. Gallagher," she defended. "It has to do with being in the Navy. His patriotic duty—oh, just ask him."

"Does he really plan to send *you* away, Mrs. Quigley?"

"He just might do that. Except—well, I think he still needs me to help with these children. Poor Jonas. He's been holding so much anger inside for so long."

"Anger at his father? At what happened to Miss Broderick?"

Griselda nuzzled her chin against the sleeping child. "You'd better ask Jonas."

Sydney moved slowly across the room and peered into a kettle. "Porridge? May I have some? I'm hungry. And maybe Keeley would enjoy some too. And while we eat, maybe you can tell me what happened to—" She couldn't bring herself to mention Abigail Broderick's name. She nodded toward the child on Griselda's lap. "He looks like Keeley."

"This is Danny, Keeley's brother."

"I gather that. Maybe you can tell me a little bit about them and why Keeley keeps running away. Perhaps I can help."

Griselda eased the sleeping child more comfortably in her arms. "I guess I owe you that much. You see, their father was one of Abigail's boys. He brought them to us a couple of weeks ago—that's the night when everything went wrong."

"The night Miss Broderick had her heart attack?"

"How did you know that?"

"Mr. Gallagher told me. That's why I flew over."

"That's right. Your mother and Abigail were old friends. No wonder you came."

Friends? More links to the past. "Yesterday when I arrived, you said you thought we needed to talk. I think this is as good a time as any."

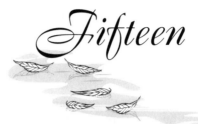

Fifteen

When Sydney opened the front door, a stranger stood on the top step. "Good morning," she said. "I was just going out."

"Then you won't mind if I come in?"

Appearing to be in his thirties, he was a pleasant-faced man and held a medical kit in his hand. He stepped inside the corridor. "I'm Dr. Wallis. How is my patient today?"

Puzzled, she said, "Your patient? I guess I didn't know anyone was ill. Well, Danny did hurt his knee, but I'm certain that Boris took all of the children down to the stables, and I'm just going out to look for Jonas."

"He won't be hard to find. He's across the river playing his bagpipes. I knew it was Jonas the minute I heard the music."

"By the way, Doctor, I'm Sydney Barrington. Would you mind telling Mrs. Quigley I won't be gone long?"

A noticeable twitch pulsated along the doctor's jaw as he returned her smile. "Are you staying at the manor?"

"Yes, and unexpectedly for several more days. I had a reservation at The Sheepfold, but when I didn't show up they gave it away. They promised to find me a room early next week—that will make it easier to make an appointment with the solicitor in town."

"Edmund Gallagher?"

"Yes. You know him?"

"Since boyhood. Have a good day, Miss Barrington."

She stood in the doorway, expecting him to turn toward the West Wing where the Admiral lived. Instead he climbed the magnificent stairs with his medical kit still in his hand. An uncanny feeling stirred inside her, leaving her certain that she already knew the answer.

Sydney left the manor and made her way back over the path she had taken yesterday. Crossing the River Windrush she climbed the hills toward the keening wail of the bagpipes. She longed to hear a march or a reel, but it was a lament that the wind carried toward her. She saw Jonas now, a towering picture of strength against the backdrop of emerald hills. She cut through a patch of wildflowers, pressing on toward the Admiral's son.

The collie lay near his master's feet, both the man and dog looking peaceful. The sudden lurch inside her was a heartbeat out of sync with Barrington Enterprises. *I could be happy here,* she told herself, and wondered where the thought had been born.

Jonas turned as she approached. The music died in the middle of the dirge. He smiled. "I wasn't certain we would meet again."

"I came up to apologize."

His sea-blue eyes twinkled. "No need."

"But I thought you were the gardener, Mr. Willoughby."

"And I thought you brought your daughter with you."

"I'm not married."

"That could be good news."

"It was foolish of me thinking you were the gardener. I had no right to interfere in your quarrel anyway."

"A man out of control needs to be checked."

Jonas, she noted, had a full, sensitive mouth, a firmly set jaw, and the tantalizing scent of a woody cologne. The pinched frown still wedged between his brows as he talked to her. In spite of their snap-judgment animosity, his features lit with an amused smile. "I garden, but I'm not a gardener. And I'm certain Griselda has told you that I'm the Admiral's son?"

"She takes a good bit of pride in that." Sydney averted his probing gaze. "Now that I'm here, I'm not sure what else to say."

"You've come too far to turn around and leave." He bent down and placed his bagpipes on a soft quilt. "I have no chair to offer, but the grass is like velvet to the touch up here."

"I can't stay long."

He pointed toward the ground. "Then be my guest for as long as you can stay. Or even longer."

Once seated, he faced her. "I'm glad you came, Miss Barrington. I was embarrassed once Griselda told me your name. I should have recognized you when you first arrived."

"Recognized me?" Surely if she had seen Jonas before, handsome as he was, she would have remembered.

"Abigail often talked about you."

"But I never met her."

"But you did. A long time ago. I didn't like it when your parents took you away—and Abigail was heartsick. You don't remember being here, do you?" he asked.

She had a feeling of floating, of drifting back in time. She tried to remember his face, his voice from the past. "I'm not sure. Vaguely, maybe. The fountain was familiar when I saw it. And walking up to the manor yesterday, I expected to see a beech tree around the first corner, with a clump of azaleas by its roots—I was wrong. I found musk orchids instead."

He smiled. "One of the gardeners dug up the azaleas after a rather nasty storm. The orchids grew wild." He tugged at a blade of grass and blew it away. "I was ten when they took you away. I thought I would never see you again."

She turned and looked into those mesmerizing eyes. "You seem so certain I was here before. Was I one of Abigail's children?"

"Only briefly—until the Barringtons took you to America. They brought you back twice when you were a little girl."

In a flash, it was clear in her mind. "I wore a pink bow in my hair. A ponytail, I think. And I blew out birthday candles."

154

"Yes. You were six that day."

She touched his hand. "But I don't remember you, Jonas. I don't remember Abigail."

"Your mother and Abigail were friends. You stayed here with Abigail for several weeks until the Barringtons adopted you."

"Then I've come back—I've come home?"

She looked back toward the stately manor where the property stretched out for miles. The immensity of it struck her.

"Have you always lived here, Jonas?"

He nodded. "My parents kept a London home, but mostly in the summers and on holidays we lived here in Stow-on-the-Woodland."

"I thought the property belonged to Miss Broderick."

He laughed. "No, it belonged to my mother. It's been in our family for generations. Several hundred years at least. My people made their fortune in the wool trade, but I don't think I would have liked my forefathers lording it over the village people, riding their hunts, eating off the fat of the land. My mother was not like that. She was warmhearted and kind; people loved her. When Mother died, I thought Dad would move us back to our London home. But I think he came to see the land as a good thing."

Her mind reeled. "Then, *you* are next in line?"

"Of course. I'm the only child. My mother's brother never wanted the place. He took over the family estate in Scotland and is content there. So with Dad ill, the burden of care is mine."

She broke off a tiny yellow flower and stared down at it. "What will you do with the property?"

"When I first came home, I talked to our family solicitor about selling it and placing Dad and Abigail in senior residences. It's much more land than we can tend to as a family. I even agreed to give the solicitor, Edmund Gallagher, the option of parceling off the land to developers if I'm away. He told me he had a buyer in mind."

Himself, she thought. "Why won't you be here, Jonas?"

He rubbed his knuckles. "I'll be back at sea. Some people think I followed in my father's footsteps, but by the time I was nine I wanted a Navy career myself." His fingers glided over his knuckles. "Now that I'm here, I realize I can't sell the place out from under him. He's an old man. He was old when I was born."

"Would you give up your Navy career?"

"The sea is my life. Yet I've spent my life trying to please my father. Selling what belonged to Mother would only hurt him."

"You should preserve the land for your own children."

He smiled. "It seems unlikely that I'll have a family."

"You're still a young man."

"But my fiancée is dead."

"I'm sorry. What happened to her?"

"An accident. A terrible accident."

Sydney envisioned a plane crash or a car careening off the motorway at a reckless speed.

"If we had married, she would have overseen the care of Broadshire Manor. Now I have to make other arrangements. The taxes are unbelievable—more than Dad or I can handle now."

She thought of Edmund Gallagher. Of the illegal maneuvers he had in mind. "Have you decided what to do, Jonas?"

"I've considered turning most of the property over to the National Trust. They acquire ancestral homes like mine. I can donate the property in lieu of taxes, maybe continue to live here if I open part of the manor to the public."

"Is that what you want to do?"

"I want to keep a piece of the land to build on. But since coming home this time, I realize it is wrong to keep this vast property for one family. My solicitor would like to own the

156

land himself. Or sell it. But too much of the money would go into his pocket, and the Willoughby name would soon be forgotten. The government would preserve our name and the integrity and beauty of this place for generations to come."

"Then you have real problems," Sydney said, picking another small flower.

She longed to be honest with him and tell him that she had come to claim her windfall from Abigail Broderick. But the manor belonged to the Willoughby family. Or had some quirk in the law left it in the hands of Abigail Broderick? If so, the Admiral's son faced the shock of his life.

"Sydney, if the National Trust takes over, I wouldn't have to worry about a staff large enough to run the manor. In the early days it took shepherds, gardeners, plumbers, domestic staff, stable boys. World War II brought a lot of changes. Some of the property was divided up, farmed by locals. The staff dwindled once Mother died. But I still remember chauffeurs driving my mother and me back and forth to London."

He faced her, looking chagrined. "I'm sorry. All I've done is talk about my land and my family. What about you? Why have you come back after all these years?"

She couldn't tell him the whole truth, but she said, "I'm here on business."

"A businesswoman! Then tell me, what would you do with the manor?"

"I'd use my money to maintain the gardens, keep a place for the children, and restore the manor to its former glory."

"A rich businesswoman. A noble aim but an impractical one. Better for the National Trust to assume the care and restoration. I think that would please my mother. But you sound like Abigail. Is that why you came? To take up her work with refugee children?"

She didn't answer him but looked off at the distant hills. Sitting high on a wold gave her a sense of splendor and grandeur, a view of the sweep and breadth of the land. She felt part of the magnificent landscape and a deep sense of security with solid earth beneath her feet, the heavens above her.

"It's beautiful here, Jonas, with the sun on the hills, the wildflowers flourishing, the sheep grazing. I'm overwhelmed with the unending beauty of the Cotswolds. Maybe that's why I came back—to soak up the beauty again."

He said solemnly, "Abigail always said this place gave her an awareness of the sovereignty of God. I tend to agree with her. The hills are always here. The color changes. The seasons change, but the hills are everlasting."

"I'm glad I came back, Jonas."

Her words pleased him. He leaned forward. "You think it is lovely now. You should see our fiery autumns. We're ablaze with color. London seems drab then."

"Perhaps I'll come back then."

"Promise?"

She flushed at his casual remark. Yes, she would come back if she knew Jonas Willoughby would be here.

Jonas liked the sensuous curve of Sydney's mouth, the teasing ripple in her laughter, the intelligence that sparked in her eyes as she listened to him. It surprised him how easy it was to talk to her, how effortless to hold her attention without turning on the old Willoughby charm. He thought of that crush he had on a little girl when he was ten. Had anything changed? Yes, she had grown into a beautiful woman, and he felt suddenly as uncertain as he had when they were children. He wanted to pursue their friendship, to delay her leaving Stow-on-the-Woodland. But did he dare allow her presence to lure him from his true purpose in the village? Could he really trust her?

She drew her legs up and encircled them with her arms. Slender wrists. Slender ankles. "It's peaceful here, like my cabin by the river. I look at a place like this and think I could stay forever."

"Stay. I'd like that."

"Randolph teases me about finding my castle in the sky."

"Competition?" he teased. "I might be a jealous man."

She laughed. "He's my right-hand man at Barrington."

"As long as he doesn't bother your left hand," he said, noting the blanched skin where a ring had been. *Stop it,* he told himself. His quick, easy way of flirting had irritated Louise. A charm he had learned from his father. But this woman—like Louise—deserved more than a brief flirtation.

He pointed back toward the west wing. "My father stays there. He's ill and frail; that's why I've come home."

"He didn't come down for breakfast this morning."

"He never comes for breakfast. Lucas—the steward who takes care of him—thinks he rests better away from others."

"And what do you think?"

"That my father will never change."

"And now you're not talking about breakfast. But why do you have him locked away in a room of his own?"

His tone sharpened. "We don't have him locked away. I told you, the Admiral's steward is with him."

"I haven't met the man, and already I don't like Lucas. Your father is a retired Admiral. That means he's spent a lifetime with people. How sad to have no friends now."

Jonas rubbed his moist palms. "Dad's a bit dotty. Confused."

"And you're ashamed of him? Don't be, Jonas. Even someone with memory loss needs to be among friends."

"Lucas takes him out on the balcony each morning. Gregor pops in once a day. More if we let him. And Abigail and I used to take turns staying with him at night. But it's up to me now." He looked directly at her. "Would you like to meet my father?"

"Yes. It sounds like Gregor adores him."

"Most people are afraid of him."

Jonas rallied the dog and hoisted his bagpipes to his shoulder. When they reached the west wing, the Admiral was sitting by the window, his steward standing beside him.

"Dad, I brought company. She's a friend of Abigail's."

The old man went on gazing out the window. "The tide's coming in. We've got to get the ship underway."

"Right-o, Admiral," Lucas said.

Lucas was an unpretentious-looking man. Tall, authoritative, visibly showing concern for the Admiral. His hair was cut short, poking up with a reddish glow. Sydney wasn't certain which man was dotty. Or were they playing a game?

Whatever they were doing, the Admiral went on with his orders. "Let's take the *HMS Barham* out today."

"Very good, sir."

"Dad," Jonas said sharply.

His father turned his hoary head to acknowledge them, suddenly aware of their presence. The Admiral's face was lined with sea wrinkles, his eyes wide, curious.

"Is that you, Willoughby?" the Admiral said. "You going with us? You don't have a command of your own. When I was your age—"

Jonas winced. "Not this time, sir. You have company."

At the scold in Jonas's voice, the old man's eyes settled on Sydney. Even at eighty he was still handsome with strong chiseled features. Thinning fluffs of black hair framed the bald spot. "Is she a snotty? And I don't want any women on my ship."

"That's a midshipman," Jonas said, embarrassed. "That's what they called them when Dad first entered the service."

"I wouldn't be very good at sea, sir. I'd be seasick."

He laughed, pleased. "I've been with the Royal Navy all my life. Did Willoughby tell you I entered the service as a cadet at Osborne in the midthirties? Joined the fleet as a midshipman eighteen months later." The dull gaze in his eyes brightened. "I was on one of those big battleships in time to give that war a run for its money. Do you remember that war, snotty?"

"I wasn't born then, sir," Sydney said.

"It's a shame you missed that war. I was given a command of my own. I wasn't like Willoughby here—turning down a ship."

"He's right on both counts," Jonas said. "Dad never turned down anything—for anyone. By war's end he was in command of a warship on escort duty in the Atlantic."

"Hunting U-boats," the Admiral said proudly.

"A remarkable career," Sydney told him.

"Lucas, we have guests. Should we have tea?" the Admiral suggested.

"Don't bother, Lucas. . . . We won't stay long, Father."

"Stay long enough to make this young snotty welcome. We should show her my medals and ships."

"Another time, Dad."

"Yes, I will come back. You can show me your ships and medals then," Sydney said reassuringly.

"Keep her to that promise, Willoughby."

The whole time the Admiral talked, Lucas kept his piercing gaze on Sydney. His face was full, his eyes provocative as he studied her. His shirt sleeves were rolled up, his collar open at the neck. His jeans were tight, his feet bare in their loafers. A man's man and he knew it. And he knew she was aware of him.

Sydney stepped back as Lucas wheeled the old man back to his bed. With strength visible in those muscled arms, he lifted the Admiral and settled him on top of the bedding. He fluffed the old man's pillows and braced him in a sitting position.

"That's good, Lucas. I was getting tired on my watch. Now where was I, young woman?" And without a pause, he went right on commanding ships from his four-poster bed.

"He's getting excitable. Should I give him his medicine early, Commander?"

"No. Wait until bedtime, Lucas."

Sydney liked the gruff old man, but she questioned his mental status. Had he been overmedicated? Or was he sim-

161

ply losing his memory? Rambling in the past? Lucas seemed protective enough, but was he smothering the Admiral?

She flushed when she realized Lucas was watching her. Lucas seemed charming enough in his own way, yet shifty-eyed. She felt uncomfortable in his presence, wondering whether he was a double-minded man in all his ways.

She was relieved when Jonas dismissed the Admiral's steward. "We'll take over now, Lucas. Give us another ten minutes."

"Very good, sir. It will give Miss Barrington more time to hear about the Admiral's ships. The walls are lined with them." He cast a sly smile Sydney's way. "I'll get the Admiral's tray."

"Jonas," she said when Lucas had gone, "you look tired. Do you plan to sit up all night with your father?"

"I have no choice. Boris filled in for me last evening. I can't ask him to do it again."

"Then let me do it. I'd feel like I was earning my keep."

"Would you really mind? What about midnight until three? I could get some good sleep that way."

"It's a done deal, Jonas."

At midnight Sydney went back to the west wing and tapped lightly on the Admiral's door. It swung back so swiftly that it startled her. Lucas stood in the shadows glaring out at her.

"I've come to sit with the Admiral."

"I could have spelled the Commander, taken his place. But you're here now."

He led her to the Admiral's bedside where the old man lay with his eyes closed, his hoary head resting against the pillows. His breathing seemed uneasy, not that of a man asleep.

"I've given the Admiral his medication. He should be fine, but if you need anyone, pull that cord. That will bring Mrs. Quigley at once. If he grows restless—or seems out of sorts—push this buzzer. It's wired to my room in the stables."

He stared down at the Admiral with an expression that could only be a mixture of respect and disdain. She had no doubt that there had once been a close friendship between the Admiral and his steward. But now? Or was Lucas fighting the loss of an old friend through illness and old age?

"Good night, sir," Lucas said. "I will be back in the morning to help you bathe and dress."

The inert man on the bed remained motionless with his eyelids closed, but Sydney had discerned a slight increase in the rise and fall of the Admiral's chest. *He's awake,* she thought. *He knows exactly what is going on in this room.*

For a second she panicked at the thought of being left alone with him and then, regaining her composure, asked, "Lucas, did Dr. Wallis think the Admiral was better this morning?"

"Dr. Wallis?"

"Yes, I met him when he came this morning."

"Dr. Wallis," Lucas said coolly, "does not take me into his confidence. Besides, he wasn't calling on the Admiral."

Her unease grew. "Should I sit by the Admiral's bedside?"

"That's what Miss Broderick always did. I don't know how the commander spends his time here." The words implied doubt, scorn. "The Admiral likes a cup of hot chocolate at one in the morning. At least he did when Miss Broderick sat with him."

"I can do that. Should I awaken Mrs. Quigley?"

"No. I keep a hot plate in the bathroom and all the fixings. I have a tin of sweet breads there as well."

With a quick nod he was gone, closing the door emphatically behind him. She listened, waiting for the echo of his footsteps to fade. Satisfied that he had gone, she reached for a chair and pulled it to the bedside.

"Abigail." The old man's eyes fluttered. He glanced around, his gaze vacant for a moment, then he focused on her. "Where's Abigail?"

Hadn't they told him what happened? Or did he forget and ask the same question over and over? "I've come in her place. Your son will be here later."

He waved his veined hand in disgust. "He should be back on *The Invincible* flying those planes of his, not here with me."

The words of a rational man, a concerned father. "He wants to be with you while you're ill."

"Ill?" he roared. "I'm not sick. I'm just an old man stuck with all the appendages of old age. Give me a cloth, girl. Whoever you are."

"I'm Sydney Barrington. I visited you earlier today."

"I don't remember. Just give me a cloth."

She handed him her handkerchief. He lifted his head from his pillows and spit into it. Pills spilled from his mouth. She took the hanky and dabbed his lips.

"It looks like you didn't take your medicine."

"A man can't think for himself with all of that forced on him. Abigail doesn't make me take that stuff when she's here. We just sit and talk." A faint twinkle touched his eyes. "And we hold hands when Lucas leaves."

Abigail's name again. Was she alive, or only alive in the old man's mind?

He looked at her with a piercing gaze. "You're an attractive young woman. Like Abigail and my wife. Did you know my wife?"

"Only through the portrait on the wall. Lady Willoughby died when I was a child. But she and Abigail were great friends."

His eyes mocked. "Were they?" he asked. "I'm tired. I'll rest now before my son gets here. And when I wake up, Miss—"

"Sydney Barrington."

"Well then, Miss Sydney, we will talk then, and you can tell me why you're here."

He sank back against his pillow and five minutes later snored peacefully. Sydney glanced again at the three pills and decided on the spur of the moment not to leave them for Lucas to discover. She wandered around the half-lit room trying to tie the enigma of the man together. She found the pill bottles in the Admiral's top dresser and made her way to the table lamp to read their labels. She matched the pills. Two sleeping pills and another medication if the Admiral became combative. She tried to make out the doctor's name, but it was not Dr. Wallis.

Anger rose inside her. A man who had been in command of ships should not be reduced to a shell of a person, in constant stupor from medication. She folded her handkerchief over the pills and tucked them into her pocket. Moments later, changing her mind, she walked into the bathroom, poured the pills into the bowl, and watched them swirl into oblivion. But she would nose around and find out why he was so heavily medicated.

"Abigail," came a voice from the dark.

She turned and hurried back into the bedroom. From the doorway she saw the outline of the Admiral's frail body lying on the monstrous four-poster bed. He was tall, but he appeared frail and uncertain in the shadows. He lifted his hand.

"Abigail," he called again.

"I'm coming," Sydney said. "And we'll have hot chocolate together."

Sixteen

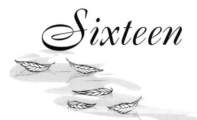

Sydney reached the solicitor's office before Edmund Gallagher arrived and stood with her back against the buff-colored building waiting for him. Above her, the green shingle swayed and creaked. Another half hour passed before a smartly attired man strode purposefully toward her.

She stepped forward. "I'm Sydney Barrington."

Gallagher's cool expression never wavered. He was younger than she had expected, perhaps still in his thirties, and looked smooth and professional in his tailored suit.

"I'm sorry I missed our appointment on Saturday, but an emergency kept me in London. I hope you didn't wait long," he said nonchalantly.

He unlocked the door and walked in ahead of her, taking precise steps. His office looked modern except for an old cloak rack where he tossed his Burberry coat. He opened the windows as he passed them, put his briefcase on the floor beside him, and pressed the button on his answering machine.

"Edmund, this is Cora Churchill. Please return my calls."

Sounds familiar, Sydney thought.

The second caller said, "This is Dr. Wallis returning your call, Edmund."

She smothered her surprise when Jeff's cheerful voice echoed in the room. "Mr. Gallagher, this is Jeffrey Van-Burien. I'm trying to reach a client of yours—Sydney Barrington. I'm on holiday at the St. Michael's vicarage in Stow-on-the-Woodland. Trust we can make contact with her there. Tell her we have some surprises for her."

Behind his thick-rimmed glasses, Edmund's cold eyes met hers. "You didn't leave a number for him to reach you?"

"I guess not. Isn't Miss Broderick buried at St. Michael's?"

"It's the only cemetery in the area. Will you be going on to Stow-on-the-Woodland today, Miss Barrington?"

She didn't tell him she had already been there. "I really should. Imagine friends from home being here at the same time."

"Imagine," he agreed. "It's not exactly a tourist spot."

"But why would they be staying at the vicarage?" *Unless they had discovered something—or someone—buried there.*

"There are no hotels. The vicar tends to take in strangers. The St. Michael's church tower will be the first thing you see from the road when you drive to the village." His eyes narrowed. "Ask for directions to the Very Reverend Charles Rainford-Simms. The church is centuries old, the cleric there not much younger."

Waving his hand at the seat across from him, he sank down into his leather chair and folded his ringed hands on the desktop. "I conclude you are here regarding Miss Broderick's will and your inheritance? I have a full schedule this morning, so we need to set up a regular appointment time. Preferably in London."

She decided to play his game. "No, preferably here where it is convenient for me. I came for the burial of my friend, Mr. Gallagher. There's no point in driving back to London."

"You are rather late for a funeral. I was unable to attend myself. I believe they cremated—"

"You said she was to be buried, per her own wishes. So it's not too late to place flowers on Miss Broderick's grave—once I know where it is."

"I may have rather disturbing news for you. There have been some legal problems. Some unexpected debts. You do remember I told you everything could be handled by my office?"

"I was coming to Europe on business anyway."

He whirled in his seat and reached for a folder from his file. "It looks now as if we must sell the property to pay the sizable debts. I'm not certain what will be left for you—perhaps a few thousand in American currency. That's one of the problems, Miss Barrington."

"What about the other six problems? The children?"

A tic twisted the corner of his mouth. "We will find proper homes for them when the time comes. And I told you on the phone that we have a prospective buyer for the property."

She challenged him. "So you still plan to sell the property and send the occupants away? Were you going to consult me first?"

"I thought we agreed on the phone—"

"I don't think we settled on anything. That's why I'm here."

"Then I assume you would like me to go ahead with that offer? It's a private arrangement, Miss Barrington."

I'm certain it is. "I would like to meet with the buyer."

He opened his mouth to speak and wiped his lips instead. "I told you, it is a private arrangement. If you can wait until Wednesday, I will arrange to drive you out to Stow-on-the-Woodland. That way we can inspect the property together."

"I have my own car. I can meet you there, but let's meet tomorrow. And I want to see the children and Mrs. Quigley. That was the housekeeper's name, wasn't it?"

"Stay away from the manor. Mrs. Quigley is a cantankerous old woman. I don't think we should trouble her right now. I need time to work out the arrangements with the buyer. He's already signed a tentative agreement with me."

You're talking about Jonas, the Admiral's son, the rightful heir. There were obvious distortions and lies in what he told her, but it was too soon to mention Jonas. She tried to guess Jeff VanBurien's counsel and said, "The buyer signed an agreement with you, Mr. Gallagher? Not with me?"

"I am Miss Broderick's solicitor. I was the obvious contact. With all the debts piling up, the final settlement could be months away. Perhaps years. There's no need for you to stay."

No need to come? No need to stay? According to Jonas, the story was different. She was certain that she had inherited nothing. Not a parcel of land, not a child. But how could she pack up and go home? How could she walk out on Keeley O'Reilly? Again this morning, the child had popped into her room, tugging at her sheet and her heartstrings. Or how could she walk out on Commander Willoughby? Wasn't it her responsibility now to make certain he inherited the property that was rightfully his?

"Will anyone else contest the will?" she asked. "According to your phone calls, I am the sole heir."

"But if there's nothing left—"

I've seen the property, Mr. Gallagher, she thought. *It's immense. And somehow I don't believe that the bill collectors are lined up at the door.*

She pitied the man sitting across from her, digging himself in deeper. Was greed driving him? Or would that legal document sitting in his folder ban Jonas from falling heir to the Willoughby property? She fixed her gaze on Gallagher's hands—large, smooth hands, the nails finely clipped. Then she met those sharp eyes again and wished she could look into his mind and heart. He was backing himself into a corner of lies.

"May I see the will?" she asked.

"It would be best—"

"Mr. Gallagher, I have only recently gone through the settlement of my parents' estate, a complicated one. I realize that wills take time, that problems arise, that debts must be paid. But as sole heir, I do have a right to review Miss Broderick's will. And I will have a right to be advised of all claims against her estate."

The tic started again. He slid the paper across the desk and tapped the place where Sydney's name was entered. "I

169

hereby will, give, devise, and bequeath all the rest, residue, and remainder of my estate. . . ."

Her name leaped from the page. Before she could read further, he pulled the file away. "Now do you believe me?"

Edmund Gallagher had told the truth. But something was still wrong. What quirk of the law had passed Broadshire Manor from Lady Willoughby to her lifelong friend Abigail—and on to Sydney?

"I want to have a copy of that will. And perhaps you have a copy of Abigail Broderick's death certificate there in your file. I'd like a copy of that as well."

Edmund's skin blanched. "Just now I cannot do as you ask. For reasons already explained, the settling of the estate has been delayed."

She wanted to laugh. What had she walked into? "Another excuse, Mr. Gallagher?" *A time-out to change your game plan?*

His face remained ashen. He spoke with subdued rage. "I have no control over the barrister's decision. You see, you may not be the rightful heir."

The truth at last. Or more lies? "Who then?"

As Edmund contemplated his next words, a smirk touched his lips. He took great pleasure in his announcement. "You may not be the sole heir. Miss Broderick may have a child of her own."

Had one of Abigail's hidden children laid claim to her estate? She had a dozen sons. Perhaps more. Sydney felt flushed. "I didn't know Abigail Broderick was married."

"I don't know the particulars. I just wanted to settle this business and not get you involved."

"But I am involved, Mr. Gallagher. And I'm more concerned than you know. Would you mind telling me again about her? About her illness? Her history? Her death? Her burial?"

Gallagher put his hands to his temples. "I need time, Miss Barrington. Don't you understand?"

"I haven't understood anything since you first called me. Something tells me that all I have inherited is trouble. But I won't run away from it. I intend to see this one through."

He bristled. Color came back to his face. The tic twisted the corner of his mouth even more. "Are you questioning my integrity?"

"Don't make the situation any worse. If Miss Broderick has a child, then I am obviously not the sole heir." Again she felt pity for Gallagher and the web he had drawn around himself. "Put your plans for developing Stow-on-the-Woodland on hold. I want to see Miss Broderick's grave before we make any decisions at all. And when we meet again, my lawyer will be at my side."

He hit the repeat button on his answering machine and listened to Jeff VanBurien's voice echoing through the room again. "Somehow I believe it will be this Mr. Jeffrey VanBurien."

"Perhaps. But don't put the manor on the selling block. I'm certain my lawyer will insist that you locate that child first, if such a child exists."

He grabbed another excuse. "It's possible that he's deceased now. No one in the village has ever heard of him."

"But you have! So make certain."

He picked up his pen. "Where are you staying?"

Sidestepping his question, she said, "I'll be in touch, Mr. Gallagher. And most definitely, the next time we meet, I will ask my lawyer to join us."

As she stepped from his office, Edmund dialed the health center. "I don't care if Wallis is seeing a patient," he said gruffly. "Get him on the line."

He didn't have to wait long.

"Edmund, don't upset my nurse like that again."

"That Barrington woman is here. She's going to be a problem for me. I can't lose that Broadshire property. You've got to help me stop her. Did you change one of the grave markers for me?"

"Of course not. And I know she's here, Edmund. In fact, I've met her. She's staying at Broadshire Manor."

Edmund cleared his voice three times before he could mumble, "Has she seen Abigail? Does she know—"

"I don't think so, but it won't take long for her to figure it out."

"I've gone too far."

"I've been telling you that, Edmund. You need to know. Miss Barrington has met the Admiral. But you have a bigger problem than the Admiral. Miss Barrington has met the Admiral's son."

When Sydney reached the village, she parked the car near the center of town and walked through the tree-lined path to the Church of St. Michael's. She found the vicar and his two guests wandering through the church cemetery.

Sydney felt an immense relief at the sight of them. Jeff was his lean, beanpole self. Her ally, her friend. She fought off the urge to run up and throw her arms around him. His brother Chan, long-legged and pleasant, was just another link to home. Chandler was the better looking of the brothers with shoulders broad enough to cry on if things got rough for her. As tall as the brothers were, the vicar towered above them; he looked like he'd bent forward most of his life— out of awkwardness in his boyhood, out of hearing loss in his older years. Yet he turned at the sound of her footsteps behind him and smiled.

"Well, here's the young woman you've been expecting. Miss Barrington, I believe. I've heard a good bit about you from Mrs. Quigley. And from Gregor. And, of course, from these friends of yours. You must visit me in the vicarage while you're here."

She was struck by the kind eyes that looked down at her and felt an immediate warmth toward Charles Rainford-

Simms. For a second, the joy in the cleric's eyes dimmed. "I was just showing the boys where my youngest daughter is buried."

Sydney glanced at the tombstone. It was old-fashioned and cut of stone but not tilted or cracked like the older monuments that lay in uneven rows. Fresh flowers had been placed on the grave.

Louise Rainford-Simms, it read.

Sydney subtracted quickly. "She was very young."

"Too young to die the way she died," her father said.

Uncomfortable at the catch in the vicar's voice, she turned to Jeff. "Jeff, I was shocked when I heard your message coming over the answering machine at the lawyer's office."

He slipped his arm around her. "And don't think we weren't surprised when you didn't show up at the bed-and-breakfast."

"We were downright worried," Chandler agreed. "If we hadn't gone back to The Sheepfold after breakfast this morning, we wouldn't have known you were safe."

"Chan's right. The owner told us she gave away your reservation when you didn't show up. We stayed there last night."

Sydney chuckled. "She probably gave you my room, but why did you leave that crazy message at Gallagher's office?"

"To let you know we were still here for you. The lady at The Sheepfold did us another favor when she steered us to the vicar."

The vicar smiled patiently. "It seems like I've had more guests lately than I've had parishioners. It will be nice to have you swell the congregation on Sunday."

"Count me out," Jeff told him.

Chan kicked him. "We'll both be there, Reverend."

Charles seemed a kindly sort with his bushy brows knit together. "It's tea time. I'll go in and ask my housegirl to make a spot of tea for all of us."

He strode off with a young man's gait, his snowy white hair thick and unruly.

"Likable old guy," Jeff said. "He knows this village well and everyone in it. I even asked him about Edmund Gallagher. He said Gallagher doesn't attend the worship services. And it seems that Gallagher's father was much more liked in the village."

"Well, after my visit with Gallagher today, I wasn't too impressed," Sydney added. "Something funny is going on. But I got a quick glance at the will. My name really is there."

"It can't be, Syd. That's what we wanted to tell you. Seems like the owner at The Sheepfold knows the Willoughby family well. She said Jonas will inherit the property when his father dies. And when I mentioned about Abigail Broderick dying, she just stared at me and said, 'Dead? She's a fighter, that one.'"

"The woman's exact words," Chan agreed. "She filled us in on the night Broderick had her heart attack. She said nothing about her dying."

Sydney wasn't certain she wanted to hear any more. Here it was the middle of spring, in an idyllic place, and a cold chill engulfed her. "What is Edmund Gallagher trying to pull?"

"His own program probably. That's another reason I called and left a message on his answering machine. I wanted him to know you had friends here in town who were looking out for you."

She gave them a quick rundown on the visit and said, "I told him that I won't return without my lawyer at my side."

"Good girl. One other thing," Jeff said. "We heard rumors about an IRA terrorist being shot—maybe dying— here in Stow-on-the-Woodland the night Broderick had her heart attack. We picked that little nugget up at The Sheepfold too."

Sydney laughed it off. "What would an IRA rebel be doing in a peaceful village like this?"

Jeff glanced at Chandler, then back to Sydney. "They believe he was one of Miss Broderick's boys."

"When we heard that, we decided to drive on to Stow-on-the-Woodland even if we had to camp out on the hills. Of course, I'm glad the vicarage turned up."

The vicar stood in the doorway now, beckoning them in.

"We've been here less than three hours," Chan said. "I like the vicar, but I don't like the sounds that come from the wall of that parsonage. It's a spooky place. Maybe it's just the housegirl banging around in the kitchen."

"Chan's right again. She doesn't really look like someone who would take up cooking and cleaning for a living. Cute though," Jeff said, grinning. "She's a poverty-struck artist, so the vicar took her in. He certainly didn't take her in for her cooking."

"I'm sure Jeff told you I'm a music critic by profession. But the notes that are playing in these Cotswold Hills, and particularly here in Stow-on-the-Woodland, are out of tune. We really want you to pack up and leave, Sydney."

She thought of Keeley and Jonas. Of the unanswered questions about Abigail Broderick and the lawyer who wanted to betray her. "I can't leave. Not yet. Not without knowing what's going on."

"I told Chan that you'd say that. That's why we're digging in at the parsonage. You stay. We stay."

Seventeen

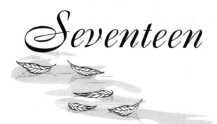

Sydney sat at Griselda's kitchen table, her mind on anything but the chatter of the children. For those few short hours on arrival, she had gloried in the prospect of taking over the manor. Now she knew the only thing she had inherited was trouble. Everything else belonged to the Admiral's son: the magnificent manor house and its gardens, the well-kept stables, and even the housekeeper who seemed lost in her own black mood this morning.

Did she dare draw Griselda into a conversation about the missing Abigail Broderick and the solicitor who hedged with the truth? Or was Abigail Broderick really dead and buried?

Sydney glanced at Keeley. Strands of the child's red hair dangled in the porridge. Her juice sat on the table untouched. Woeful eyes met Sydney's. What was behind the unhappiness there?

"Honey, you need to eat," she said.

Keeley slapped the porridge with her spoon, her lower lip trembling. "I'm not hungry."

"Do you want me to help you eat?" Sydney offered.

"Let her alone. She knows the rules in Griselda's kitchen."

Keeley's tears fell into her porridge bowl. Sydney tried again. "Mrs. Quigley, after Keeley finishes eating, I could take all of the children for a walk down by the Windrush."

"That'd be good of you."

It looked like a long standoff between the housekeeper and Keeley. Sydney kissed the top of Keeley's head. "Finish your breakfast, sweetheart, and then we'll go for a walk."

Griselda glared at them both. "Promise her a ride on that pony Lucas keeps for her and you'll get further. You do ride, don't you?"

"Yes, and well. Is there a horse I could ride?"

"Of course. Ask Lucas."

As she left the room, Sydney wondered whether the children would consider it a game if they explored the cemetery in search of names. She wanted to find the Willoughby and Broderick family plots. Gregor would know exactly where to take her, but finding Abigail's gravestone, if one existed, had to be casual.

She closed the kitchen door behind her and almost bumped into Lucas carrying an empty tray back to the kitchen. "Good morning. How's the Admiral?"

"Getting ready to ship out as usual. This morning he thinks the bedroom is the bridge of the *Queen Elizabeth*. He sailed on that great lady once."

"Lucas, I'd like to go riding with Keeley tomorrow."

"Boris can saddle the horses for you if I'm busy. I'll mention it to him."

She stood in the corridor for a few seconds as he entered the kitchen. Except for the room where she was staying, the other rooms on the east wing were ghostly apparitions shrouded in dustcovers. She would like to search them all, but she would have to wait until everyone retired. Last evening she had gone to the elegant dining room and later to the library to browse through the hundreds of books on the shelves. There was grandeur to every room, and the library held art treasures and portraits of Abigail's children.

Now she felt drawn back to the library where the narrow windows looked out on the hills and the Windrush. She imagined that this room was one where Abigail Broderick spent many of her hours. She saw again the quaint desk with its pigeonholes stuffed with envelopes. The day planner lay open on the desk as though Abigail had just this moment been called from the room.

Leaving the library, Sydney climbed the elegant stairwell to the second floor—and just in time to avoid Lucas's watchful eye, for she heard his booming voice as he left Griselda.

The hallway on the second floor was wide and carpeted with an Oriental runner. She tried doors and peered in. One was obviously the schoolroom where Jonas and the others had sat at the tiny desks. She wondered whether Jonas had ever gone to the primary school in the village, or had he always been sent away to boarding schools? But there were toys here too. Books and games. Perhaps they once belonged to Jonas.

Four doors led off from the schoolroom. She tried each one, finding the children's bedrooms as she did so. One had to be Gregor's with model planes on the worktable and boys' things cluttering the bed. The next room had pink comforters and frilly dolls on both beds. The third room lay empty; the fourth was obviously set up for the three smaller boys with pillows marked with their names: Danny, Yasmin, Philip.

Sydney went on prowling, room after room, delighting in the old furnishings and the thirteenth-century frescoes that reminded her of the artwork from the town of Assisi. As she stepped from one room, she saw an elderly woman inching along the hallway in bare feet. The woman was clothed in a sheer dressing gown and was bracing herself with her tissue-thin hands on the wall.

"Who are you?" Sydney asked, fairly certain that this was Dr. Wallis's patient.

The older woman's response was peppery. "I'm Abigail Broderick. Who else?"

Sydney's eyes opened wide. "Abigail Broderick? I don't know what to say. I was going down to the St. Michael's Cemetery in a few minutes to look for your grave. I thought you were dead."

"Not exactly, my dear." She poked at the shimmering gray hair hanging loosely at her neck. "I may look a wreck, but I'm quite alive. So, who are you?"

"I'm Sydney Barrington."

A sparkle lit the lined face. "You did come! I wanted you to come, dear girl. Prayed that you would."

She began to chuckle and then sobered at once. "Did someone tell you I was buried at St. Michael's?"

"Someone wanted me to believe that."

She smiled. "Mr. Gallagher, no doubt. He's always so solicitous about my welfare. Give me your hand, dear, and take me back to my room before I fall."

She leaned hard against Sydney. "Let's not tell Edmund that you've seen me. The poor man is counting on me dying." She started to chuckle again. "If I go on living—and right now I must—he will be so disappointed."

"You don't seem to trust him—so why are you laughing?"

She sighed as she sat on the bed. "He thought I wouldn't live long enough to change my will, and I intend to fool him."

"Where were you going, Miss Broderick, when I found you?"

The smile turned sad. "I was foolish enough to think I could get down the stairs without Griselda catching me."

"You're too weak to manage the stairs alone. Please don't try that again. If you want something, I'll go get it."

"You're right. My heart is fluttering, but I wanted to see the Admiral and check on Conon's children to know they were all right. No one tells me a thing. They think my heart will go wild with knowing. It's almost quit beating with not knowing."

Conon's children? Keeley? Danny? "Abigail, they're all well. Let me go down to the kitchen and get you something hot to drink. Then we can talk about a visit to the west wing."

"And you can tell me why you came back."

Sydney did a light dance down the stairs and burst into the kitchen where a smoky haze rose from the oven. Griselda stood with a hot baking dish in her hands.

"Is something wrong, Sydney?"

"There's someone upstairs who needs a hot bowl of soup."

"And who might that be?"

"Miss Broderick."

The dish in Griselda's hand crashed to the floor. "What were you doing up there?"

"Snooping around. I came here because I was told Abigail Broderick was dead. And, Mrs. Quigley, I have no intention of leaving until I know what's going on—and who these children are."

"You had no right to go up there."

"Didn't I? I've been lied to and brought over here on false pretenses. Did you know I was told I had inherited this property? That would give me every right to wander through it. But the woman hasn't even died yet. And Jonas has no idea why I'm here. He expects to take over this property when his father dies."

Griselda plopped down in a chair. "I know. The whole sorry mess is too much for all of us. Give me a minute and I'll heat some chicken broth. Abigail likes little biscuits with her soup and hot tea, so I'll send those along. But don't forget, you promised to take the children for a walk. They're waiting for you in the primrose garden."

"Oh, I had forgotten. Give me another twenty minutes."

She crept back up the magnificent stairway, walking slowly so the soup wouldn't spill. Before she touched the knob to Abigail's room, she felt a restraining grip on her wrist.

Jonas Willoughby towered above her, his face clouded. "What do you think you're doing here?"

"I'm taking a tray to Abigail—and you're hurting my arm."

He released her. "Dr. Wallis doesn't encourage visitors."

"Abigail shouldn't be cooped up here all alone."

"I plan to visit her. And Gregor comes. And Griselda spends the evenings with her after the children are in bed."

"And do you laugh with her?"

Jonas glared back. "We try not to excite her. She had a heart attack recently."

180

"I know. I heard she was dead, and she isn't. Now, Jonas, the soup is getting cold."

"Wait. I've just come from talking to Edmund Gallagher."

"That must have been an enlightening visit."

"He says you're trying to buy the property while Abigail is ill so you can parcel it out to developers. You can't do that."

"So now Gallagher is spinning lies about me. Jonas, I own a defense empire. I don't need this property—or want the headaches that go with it."

He still blocked her entry. "Do you deny meeting Edmund?"

"I don't deny anything, nor am I obligated to explain anything to you. Besides, Commander Willoughby, I understand you're back in town to track down an Irish terrorist. And they tell me he's one of Miss Broderick's children. Is Abigail aware of what you're doing?"

The smile began at the corner of his mouth. "I live here, remember? And yes, there are rumors in the village. You are well informed."

She shrugged. "Why don't we start over and work together?"

He turned the knob and pushed the door open. Abigail sat propped in her bed, her silver hair shining. She put down her hairbrush. "Jonas, dear! When did you get back from Northwood?"

"A few days ago."

"And you've been ignoring me? At least you met Sydney. Oh, dear, I can see by the pair of you that the rich American executive and the country squire have marked their battle lines. But hold off on the war. Come in. Sit with me."

"I'll come back. I'll go see how Dad is while you eat."

A sparkle came into her face. "Give him my love."

"You'll soon be well enough to see him yourself."

"Not if she has to climb up and down that staircase. Jonas, why can't we move Abigail downstairs to the room next to mine? Then she can see everyone. She could even have her meals with the rest of us."

He scowled. "I want to keep the east wing closed off."

Abigail protested. "It's been far too long, Jonas. Tell Griselda that I want to be moved down there beside Sydney. You'll do that, won't you, Jonas? The first room is the nicest."

"It was intended for someone else."

"I know. For Louise—someone who can never occupy it. Louise wouldn't want that room to remain unoccupied forever."

An hour later Sydney gathered the children to her and walked leisurely down the hillside to St. Michael's. She half expected to find a grave with Abigail's name on it, perhaps a crude marker—one more attempt on Edmund's part to deceive her.

When she opened the gate to the churchyard, Gregor made faces. "What'cha going in there for?"

"To look around. I thought we could play a little game and then we'll go on to Veronica's Tea Shoppe and have some treats."

"All of us? Philip and Danny always make a mess."

"I don't think Veronica will mind." She herded them into the cemetery and led them along the crooked rows. "Gregor, I want to find where the Willoughbys and the Brodericks are buried, so let's see how many names we can find."

"The little ones can't read," Gregor said.

"But you and I can. So let's do it?"

"That's no fun."

"I agree with the boy," Jeff said coming up behind them and startling Sydney. "Hey, kids. See that far wall? I want you to run for it, and the first one back gets some sweets."

"I'll win!" Gregor announced.

"Then we'll give the small fry a running start."

As Gregor dashed after Danny and Philip, Jeff pulled Sydney aside. "Cancel your game with the kids. We've already checked it out," he said cheerfully. "We've been over every tombstone and know the people of Stow-on-the-Wood-land for decades back. There are several unmarked graves—or stones where the lettering has been worn thin with the years—but no fresh graves. If your Miss Broderick is dead, she isn't buried here."

"You're right and I'm not looking any longer, Jeff. I found her."

"You mean—" he cleared his throat. "You mean she's buried somewhere else?"

"She's not buried at all. She's been ill, but Abigail Broderick is very much alive." Sydney laughed. "Oh, close your mouth, Jeff. I'm not making it up. It's true."

He shook his head. "You mean, the woman's really alive. Then we've been taken for a ride!"

"And I'm fighting back. Now I'm trying to find out how far Edmund Gallagher would go to deceive me."

He cocked his head. "You mean some extreme measure like replacing a grave marker so he could pretend it was Miss Broderick's?"

"Something like that."

"There are some Brodericks buried here. Abigail's parents, perhaps. Syd, I've talked to Reverend Rainford-Simms. He won't openly condemn the lawyer. It's not in him to run another man down. But he assures me there have been no fresh graves here in the last month."

"I just wish I knew what Gallagher is up to—and whether Miss Broderick is safe."

"I intend to find out, Sydney."

The children were flying back to them, Gregor doing leapfrogs over the crumbling stones. Danny tried desperately to mimic him. "We'll end up with another scraped knee," she said.

Keeley slipped her hand in Sydney's.

"Cute kid," Jeff said.

"Too young for you."

Chandler came over the cobbled walk, smiling. "Jeff is waiting for you to discover what a great guy he is, Sydney. In the meantime, he has his eye on Kersten. He thinks all artists are romantics."

"Like you, I have good taste, little brother."

"Any word on your wife, Chandler?" Sydney asked.

"She's still in Rome—although I couldn't reach her by phone last night. But I'm certain she'll be home soon."

Eighteen

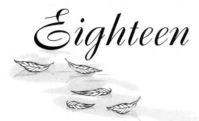

Days later, Abigail smiled as she sat down on the white bench beside Sydney. "I've been watching you, my dear. Day after day. I see you are drawn to this fountain as I have always been."

"Abby, I feel so peaceful sitting here."

"The father of one of my boys sculpted it for me—his thank-you for caring for his son during a crisis time in his own life."

"There's such simplicity, such beauty to it."

"I know. Whenever I am tired or discouraged I come here and find comfort in this marble fountain with its two carefree children carved in ivory. It reminds me of all of my children. The ones who still keep in touch. The ones who never call anymore. At one time or another, every one of the children sat here with me."

"Were they in trouble?"

"Sometimes just troubled. We'd sit together and talk and pray. It's peaceful with the water spewing in ribbons of color."

"It seems sad to have such a magnificent work of art out here in this tiny hamlet where so few ever see it."

"But the few who do find great pleasure. Santos's father is a well-known Italian designer. I met Victor at Dunkirk and owe my life to him. Later, when he needed someone to care for his son, he turned to me. The fountain was a gift of gratitude for taking care of Santos and, perhaps, for what might have been."

"Was Victor in love with you?"

"He was charming, but I did not love him. Later he married a beautiful Italian girl from Rome who saw his creative genius. And that was best. He would never have been happy here. Sydney, you may not remember it, but you met Victor when the plans for the fountain were drawn up." She placed her thin hand over Sydney's. "Victor chose you and Jonas as his models because he knew how special you both were to me."

"You knew me that long ago? Did you know my birth parents?"

"Just your mother, Dulcie. She was a sweet girl—beautiful and visionary. And once she met Joel, her destiny was settled."

Abigail sat pensively for a moment, then she went inside to the hall table and rummaged through the drawer. With sudden recall, she pulled a photo from beneath the blotter. She waved it triumphantly as she walked slowly back to Sydney. "Here. This was taken at Mont Blanc. That's Millicent beside me. And Kathryn—and Dulcie."

"I have that exact same picture. You were lovely, Abigail."

"Were?" she teased. "The four of us had wonderful times that summer before Dulcie met your father. We were all so young—out to conquer the world." Abigail blew the dust from the photograph and touched each face. "One of the last times I saw Dulcie was a week before they left for Africa."

"Sometimes I think I remember my parents crying and screaming as the rebels ran them out of town, down to the river. I think my mother thrust me into the arms of someone else for safety. And then the quiet. The terrible quiet."

"How could you know that, my dear? You were ten months old."

"Maybe I just want to remember."

Or maybe, Abigail thought, *you overheard that heated discussion between the Barringtons and myself when you were six.*

Aaron had insisted that the past be done with. That Sydney was his child. He would raise her without ever telling her that her parents gave up promising careers for mission-ary endeavors. Did she know that Aaron condemned the foolishness of missionaries dying as martyrs, the foolishness of risking a baby's life?

Sydney broke their silence. "We, the Barringtons that is, were never a religious family."

"Aaron wanted it that way. He and Millicent were raised differently. I worried about it when they married. Later, when they adopted you, I argued with Aaron. I told him your parents would want you raised in the church. He didn't agree."

"Dad always did what he wanted to do, patterned his own life, set his own rules, and his rules included Mother and me."

"Sydney, they didn't come back to visit me often, but your parents were generous. They set up a Swiss account for my work with the children. That Broadshire Account proved a lifesaver so many times. I was able to have the whole electrical system here rewired and the plumbing repaired."

Sydney thought of the file marked "Broadshire Account" and the controversy it had stirred back home with Randolph. Now she felt a warmth toward her father. A pleasant surprise. "Abby, after Dad died we tried to identify the Broadshire Account and never could. The Swiss banks are notoriously tight-lipped. It particularly irritated Randolph Iverson, one of my staff."

"The gentleman who calls here?"

Abigail noticed Sydney's embarrassed nod and glanced back at the photograph. "Sydney, Millicent was one of my best friends when we were younger. I hated losing touch with her. I think the money was her way of saying 'I still love you.' If only she had brought you back to see me again—"

"Mother talked about bringing me back to England. She wanted me to see where Dulcie was born and baptized. Where she married."

"Then she did plan to come back. Dulcie and Joel were married at St. Michael's. You'll find their names in the registry there."

Abigail spanned her fingers. "Charles is good about maintaining the church records. Marriages and baptisms. Births and deaths. It won't be long before he records my name there."

"Don't talk like that."

"If I don't, I'm only pretending. But what will happen to the children after I'm gone? Jonas won't want the responsibility. I was surprised when he came back to help his father. Sir James—Tobias—was a good man, but his mind-set and plans for his son were unwavering. He wanted to mold Jonas in his own likeness."

"They should be friends. Jonas followed in his footsteps."

"Like Tobias, Jonas grew up on the River Thames, cut his holiday time along the Windrush, and battled the angry sea off Cornwall." She rubbed her eyes. "I don't think the Admiral ever realized how much his son did to try to gain his love. Poor Jonas. He knew from the time he was six that Tobias expected him to carry on the family tradition as a Navy officer. But Jonas came to want it for himself by the time he was eight or nine."

"So he's married to the Royal Navy," Sydney said.

"That's part of the tradition. But he was engaged once."

"I know, but he won't talk about his fiancée."

"He's not been the same since her death. Did he never tell you her name or how she died?"

"No—just that it was a terrible accident."

"Louise is buried in St. Michael's Cemetery."

In a whisper, Sydney asked, "Reverend Rainford-Simms's daughter?"

"Yes. She was killed three years ago in an IRA bombing in Ireland. Now you can understand why Jonas is struggling with how deeply he feels about you. Wondering whether he should. The thought of getting close to someone again is too threatening."

Down the hillside, the chortling Windrush whistled through the rushes. "I used to take you and Jonas down there and let you wade in the water and chase the swans. You made such good playmates. Jonas was protective of you because he knew what had happened to your parents. Now, perhaps, it is time for you to help him."

That evening Sydney found solace on the bank of the Windrush, listening to the rippling river. Coming to the Cotswolds had become part of her search for herself, part of her search for peace. But she was pleased when Jonas came to sit with her.

"I wondered where you were, Sydney. Do you come here often?"

"Yes, with Keeley."

"I'm glad she isn't with you this time."

"Would you send her away?"

"No, but I'm glad for the chance to be alone with you." He tugged at a weed. "Don't bother with her, Sydney. She's trouble."

"She's troubled. That's what matters to me. Why does she annoy you so? She's only a little girl, Jonas."

"A little girl with an IRA terrorist for a father."

"Is *he* the man you're searching for? I don't think of Conon as a terrorist, Jonas. I think of him as Keeley's father."

"He's much more dangerous. I want to be with you, yet when we talk, we don't understand each other, do we?"

"I'd like to hear your side of the story."

"And I wish I understood why you spend so many hours on phone calls and take so many trips to the Tyne. Now Abigail tells me you've bid for another shipyard in Italy."

"I have. But if I win that bid on the British aircraft carriers, I'll build them at the Jarrow plant. And I expect to build them. You might sail on one of my ships someday, Jonas."

She saw his profile in the shadows—strong, determined, introspective. "The fleet has slimmed down," he said. "That means the ships afloat have to be the best, Sydney."

"If my company wins, they'll be the best. I do a good job the first time around. It's what my father expected of me."

"It sounds like we both had strong-willed fathers. All my life, I had everything, except my father's approval. The best schools. The best training at Gordonstoun and Dartmouth. I was good in sports. Excelled academically. But always I sought to escape the shadow and displeasure of my father."

She pictured a dark-haired boy growing up along the Thames, holidaying in the Cotswolds. Risking his life off the shores of Cornwall. Going to boarding schools. A lonely boy; a distant father; a dead mother. "My parents adored me," she said. "They gave me everything. Even the things I didn't know I wanted."

"We were both fortunate. Gregor on the other hand has nothing. Everything he once had is gone. I have plans for Gregor. Boarding school at Gordonstoun. Then Dartmouth and the Navy."

"Is that what Gregor wants?"

"Gordonstoun is a good boarding school, if he can qualify. I went when I was eight."

"It's tradition with you. But you didn't have your life torn apart by a war. You didn't lose your whole family."

"My mother died when I was young."

"Yes, I know, but there was always someone here for you. You were never totally alone. Jonas, don't think by arranging for his financial needs and schooling that you've discharged your duty. You made a pact with that child the day you put your arm around his shoulders and allowed him to walk to the river with you and to bring the sheep in."

"I think it best to send him to my school. Prince Charles went there. So did I. I can sign Gregor up for Gordonstoun. The Navy may be more difficult since he wasn't British born. Gregor tells me if I adopt him, he won't be foreign born. But he would need a mother too."

In the distance, the church bell rang. "Do you attend the services there at St. Michael's, Jonas? Gregor does."

"I did as a boy. But not lately."

She had stirred something deep inside of him and veered away. "I shouldn't pry—but I must ask about your father. Why is he on so much medication? He falls asleep in his soup bowl."

"He was eighty his last birthday."

"It doesn't mean he has to sleep all the time."

"Lucas insists that the medication keeps him calm. He goes into London every three weeks to pick up Dad's refills."

"Why don't you have Dr. Wallis check him over?"

"Are there any other problems you'd like to solve? I moved Abigail down by your room. Now you want to play doctor with Dad."

She blushed and was glad that in the dark he didn't know. "I'm sorry. I'm like my father—good at giving orders. Dad was a blustery, outgoing man. My mother was mellow, but after thirty years of marriage she still blushed when Dad kissed her."

"And now you're alone in the world."

"You're alone when you fly in your Sea Harrier."

"But Abigail tells me that God flies with me. What about you, Sydney? Does God fly with you?"

"I guess so. I made it safely to England this time." Quickly she said, "Jonas, tell me more about your life as a pilot. Abigail says you have every opportunity to aim for the highest rank in the Navy. Is that true?"

"Anything's possible."

And he was off, telling her about his plans for the Admiralty. She competed with him, boasting about the aircraft carriers that she would build for him.

"Sydney, never have I met a woman like you—blessed with all the feminine wiles yet so abreast with the defense industry and its needs. So many women are interested in the glory of the ships coming into port—the excitement of them setting out to sea. But you want to build them. I just wish you didn't take so many trips to that shipyard. The children miss you when you're gone."

But do you? she wondered.

She couldn't tell in the semidarkness whether he was mocking her or pleased with her. Was he comparing her to someone in his past? Someone who had not measured up? He grew animated as he spoke of flying at high speeds and landing on a moving deck. She sensed something else. He was saying words, but from his expression he seemed more aware of her eyes. Her lips. Her nearness.

"Why are you here?" he asked.

"I have my father's international corporation to run."

"But why are you *really* here?"

She wanted to be honest, totally honest with Jonas Willoughby. "Because I feel at home in England, Jonas."

"Then stay."

Suddenly she was in his arms and he was kissing her softly, there by the Windrush. When he released her, she said breathlessly, "What was that for?"

"Because I really want you to stay."

Nineteen

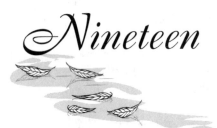

Sydney couldn't remember when the decision was made to cancel her reservation at The Sheepfold and accept Abigail's invitation to stay on as a guest at the manor. So comfortable had she become that she went freely into the kitchen for tea with Griselda. They sat there now by the old oak table with steaming cups of tea in their hands watching the children play outside.

"Keeley never plays with the others," Griselda said. "All she wants to do is go horseback riding with you."

"I promised her we'd go for a longer ride today."

"You'll be using Jonas's horse then? Maybe you and Jonas should go horseback riding together. You could pull him back into the world of the living. He knows those hills better than anyone."

"Oh, Griselda, Jonas is too preoccupied for pleasure."

"You know why, don't you? He has his mind set on finding him a terrorist. Prowls around here like as though Abigail and I have hidden the man here in Broadshire Manor. Jonas grew up under my thumb. I don't like him acting that way toward us."

"You don't make being with Jonas very appealing."

She hadn't fooled Mrs. Quigley. Griselda snorted in her impatient way. "That's up to you, Sydney Barrington. I thought you were more of a fighter. You like those Cotswold Hills out there? So did Jonas's mother. So we all do. Jonas should be showing you around. After all, you're our guest."

"I'm more of a bother to Jonas."

"Then it's up to you to make yourself visible. He can't go on grieving for Louise the rest of his life."

Griselda glanced out the window again and smiled as Gregor tossed the ball to Danny. "Gregor is good with the younger children. It's hard to remember how frightened he was when Abigail brought him here. He wouldn't let her out of his sight. Then Jonas came home and the boy was drawn to him like a magnet."

She turned her troubled gaze back to Sydney. "What do you suppose will become of Gregor once Jonas goes back to sea?"

"Jonas plans to send him to Gordonstoun."

Griselda's cup clattered as she put it back on the saucer. "Gregor isn't ready for the rigors of boarding school. Jonas even has it in the boy's head to join the Royal Navy someday. I hope Jonas gets some sense in that handsome head of his. He thinks Her Majesty's Navy is the answer to everything."

"Isn't it?" Sydney teased.

"If he wants to treat him like a son, he'd likely have to adopt the boy, and that's best done with two parents," she said with a twinkle. "I'm sure you'd be interested in that, Sydney."

Before Sydney could blame the blush on the hot tea, someone put a heavy hand on the door knocker. "I'll get it, Griselda. I was going outside to join Abigail anyway."

"I'll bring you both some tea and crumpets—we just have to get some weight back on that dear woman."

Sydney's heart beat in tune to the tapping of her heels on the long corridor. She swung the door back and looked up into the face of an attractive stranger. Everything about him seemed daring, from the disheveled strands of shiny black hair falling over his forehead to his generous mouth with its full fleshy lips. His jacket and shirt were obviously Italian, as he was.

He arched his brow at a rakish angle. "*Buon giorno,* pretty lady. I'm looking for Miss Abigail. Are you her nurse?"

"No, a friend. But Abigail isn't well enough for visitors."

"But I have come from Rome just to be with her."

She expected piercing black eyes, but when he whipped off his dark glasses they seemed more hazel, almost transparent.

"I am Santos," he announced. "Son of Victor Garibaldi. Tell her I am here. I am certain Abigail will see me. Where is she?"

"In the front garden by the fountain."

"My father's fountain! Let me surprise her."

"The excitement may be too much for her heart, Santos."

"I won her heart a long time ago." He was swiftly past her, making his way toward the glass doors. She followed and reached the garden in time to see Abigail's face bathed in a smile.

Abigail held out both hands. "Did Victor come with you?"

He took her hands and kissed her on both cheeks. "You can only take one Garibaldi at a time. But Father will come if you need him. He has just married again, for the third time, a much younger woman so she will not die on him this time. But, alas, I think he still searches for someone like you."

"Dear man. But why your surprise visit, Santos?"

"Boris called me. He said you had a second heart attack."

"The first one was only a flutter."

"Boris was afraid someone would steal the art treasures if something happened to you. That's why I am here."

"Sit down. Let me look at you."

"I am as handsome as ever. And you, dear lady, are still beautiful. Father will be pleased."

They sat sideways on the bench, their faces animated, intense. Talking. Laughing. Going happily back to the days when Santos was a child. Sydney sat near them, invited to do so, and wondered whether Abigail was aware of Santos's extraordinary charm. Or was she simply remembering the boy he had been?

They spoke of happier, lighter times. "Abigail, I think the fountain is one of my father's best works of art."

"I have few to compare it to. Sydney was one of his models."

"Ah," he said, his tantalizing gaze back on Sydney. "My father will be delighted to know that you have grown so lovely."

He took Abigail's hands again and held them. "When I was a boy I was spoiled. But you took my hands in yours—as I hold yours now—and told me that one day I would do great things."

"Have you, Santos?"

"I cannot sculpt with my father's skill. And for years, in spite of the education my father gave me, I took life lightly. But three years ago, the girl I loved would not have me. I let her go, thinking she would come running back to me. She didn't. She married someone else."

"I'm sorry."

"Don't be. Jillian is extremely happy, and I am happy for her. Because of what happened, I began to grow up. I renewed my interest in art restoration and went back as an apprentice. And, Abigail, I am good at it. That's why I'm here."

She eyed him curiously. "Something tells me you want to restore the paintings in the library?"

"Would you let me start there? Father will send others to work with me."

Her sparkle faded. "I'm not certain what will happen here. Jonas speaks of putting the property under the National Trust."

His dark face clouded, then brightened at once. "Then you will put in a good word for me with the National Trust?"

"Go, let Griselda know you are here. She can get your room ready and set a place at the table for you. I know you're anxious to go to the library and the drawing and tapestry rooms. And don't slide down the banister and break your wrist again. You'll need both hands if Jonas wants you to stay and help out."

"Father says I can work for a shingle over my head and pasta in my stomach. He will support me. It is his way of paying you back for taking care of me."

196

"Wasn't the fountain enough?"

"Father doesn't think so. He was so afraid I would not get here in time. And here you are in our favorite spot."

There was a fresh glow on her face as he left. "I have never seen you happier, Abigail," Sydney said.

"I am always happy when I see one of my children succeed."

And to hear about his father, Sydney thought.

As they sat there, Keeley ran up to them and rested her head on Sydney's arm. "You promised to take me riding on my pony."

"Oh, Abigail, will you be all right alone?"

"Go, dear. I won't be alone for long. Santos will be back, once he prowls through the manor and sees his art treasures."

"Do you think he can restore luster to the paintings?"

"If he's half as gifted as Victor, yes. He lacked confidence as a boy. But he's changed. I can see that already."

A spark of Abigail's enthusiasm rubbed off on Sydney. "It will be good for you to have Santos here when Jonas leaves."

"And when *you* leave. You are both growing restless."

I'm restless all right, Sydney thought. *But it's Jonas who has caused my unrest.*

"You're certain it's all right if Keeley and I leave? We could wait with you until Santos gets back."

"Run along, dear. You worry too much about me. I've spent many hours alone just sitting here thinking about my children."

About Santos and Jonas. And Conon O'Reilly and his children. And all the others that Sydney didn't know.

Keeley peered around Sydney. "You can watch us ride." She pointed toward the hills, far beyond St. Michael's. "We're going up there today. Sydney promised me."

"Don't let anything happen to her," Abigail cautioned Sydney. "I—I promised her father that I would take good care of her."

197

Impulsively, Sydney leaned down and kissed Abigail's cheek and tasted the salty tears falling there. "You're all right?"

Abigail turned away. "Go, please. The child needs you."

Keeley chatted happily as they left the garden and made their way to the stables. As they walked, Sydney said, "Keeley, I wish you would spend more time with Miss Abigail. She's very fond of you and Danny."

Keeley's eyes grew wide. "No, she sent my papa away."

Chilling thoughts gripped Sydney. Did Abigail send Keeley's father away? Or had she risked hiding him within the walls of Broadshire Manor in one of the closed wings or in the old keeper's cottage out by the water tower? She'd been ill for almost a month now, not well enough to hide anyone. But would she ask someone else to hide one of her boys? Boris or Mrs. Quigley, or Lucas perhaps? Sick as Abigail had been, she was still mistress of the manor. The one who gave the orders. The one who made decisions.

Or had she turned to Reverend Rainford-Simms? They often chatted about the children over cups of tea and freshly baked scones. And she always sought his advice about the cleansing of her soul, if for nothing else. Hadn't he spent a lifetime reaching out to the lost? But Charles, dear man that he was, moved about in his own world—tending his garden, enjoying his train set, wandering over the golden hills of Stow-on-the-Woodland, singing, praying. A man of the cloth! An honorable man. Would he really break his vows to the church and his parishioners and take in a castaway—even for Abigail?

She felt a nudge. "Are you sad, Sydney?"

"Just a little. But it's a wonderful day for riding."

"Can we go every day?"

"We'll see, but someday soon I have to pack up and go home."

Pack up? Leave? Go back to her responsibilities at Barrington Enterprises? How could she run out with so many things unsettled here? Randolph Iverson constantly phoned and wrote, begging her to come home, insisting that there were decisions that only she could make. Randolph rarely gave her breathing space, but it was Jonas Willoughby who took her breath away.

She felt the warmth of Keeley's hand tugging her own. "When you go, Sydney, will you take me with you?"

In her busy, workaday world, there was no room for a child. "You need to stay with Danny. He's happy here. He needs you."

"I want to be with you."

She touched the child's cheek. "I won't be able to take you with me. I'm sorry, Keeley."

She pulled back the doors to the stables and Keeley ran ahead, crying. Sydney stopped at Windstar's stall to wipe her own tears dry. She wondered if Jonas had named the stallion for a battleship, the horse was so feisty; her own thoughts were as wild and unsettled as the stallion's.

The creaking of steps snapped her attention back to the moment. She glanced to the top of the wooden staircase that led to Lucas's quarters and saw Keeley with her hand on the doorknob.

"Keeley O'Reilly, what are you doing up there? Come down this instant. We're going riding."

"I want Lucas to put me on my pony."

"I can do it this morning. Please."

"No, Lucas smells like my papa."

And what was that supposed to mean? Did Lucas smell like horses or a long day at work in the barn? She tried to recall whether he wore cologne, or did that enigma of a man with his muscular physique and brawny chest ever bother with scents?

Keeley stood on tiptoe, turning the high knob into Lucas's room. "Keeley, Lucas has gone into London to buy the Admiral's medicine. You must not go into his room when he isn't here."

"Dr. Wallis has medicine. He brings Abigail's."

Sydney tried to squash her own doubts about Lucas. "Lucas likes time away from the manor to meet with old shipmates."

The Admiral's last posting had been to the Admiralty in London where Lucas had continued as the Admiral's steward. Surely he had numerous friends in the city, even the wrong friends.

Sydney started up the wooden steps, listening to them creak, feeling the wobbly instability of the handrail. "Honey, you can't go in there when he's not home. He'll have fits if he finds you."

"What's a fit?"

"Oh, never mind. Just come down."

She extended her hand, the riding stick in the other. Keeley shrank away from her. "Oh, Keeley, I'm not going to use the stick on you. Don't you understand? I love you."

The words startled them both. Still the red curls bobbed in defiance, but when she reached the top step, Keeley flung her arms around Sydney's neck. "I want my papa," she wailed.

"I know you do. I'm glad that Lucas is good to you."

"He smells like rain."

Rain on a tweed jacket or woolly sweater? A familiar odor to Keeley. A remembered closeness to her father. Her father must have held Keeley tightly, as she was doing now, protecting her from the fear of a storm. So Lucas didn't smell of spice or a woodsy cologne but of nature's fury drenching his clothes—leaving them smelling of mildew, a scent familiar to the child.

"Was it raining the day your daddy went away?" she asked.

"I don't know."

She must ask Mrs. Quigley if it rained the day of Abigail's heart attack. That way Conon's name would be kept out of the conversation. She rocked the child, sitting on the top step and not wanting to let her go. Ever. Had they both been brought to this village for this purpose, for this moment in time to comfort each other? Sydney couldn't rock away the hurts that were deep inside the child. She couldn't even shake off her own. She missed her parents and felt a sudden rage at Conon O'Reilly and then a mixture of pity and concern. What had driven him away? What foolishness had forced him to leave his children behind?

"Let's go riding, Keeley, before it gets too late."

She set Keeley down, and the child kicked the door open and bounded into Lucas's room. A faint musty odor assailed Sydney as she followed her into the cold, cluttered room. She stared at the elaborate computer system on the L-shaped desk, a scanner and two printers attached to it. The personal furnishings seemed insignificant in comparison: a narrow, unmade bed; a chest of drawers and television set; an easy chair and a rack with socks and undershirts drying on it. The bookshelves were stocked with printer paper and boxes of computer discs.

Keeley flew to the corner of the room. "Sydney, come look at Lucas's radio."

It was not an ordinary radio. There were numerous dials and a transmitter and sending set. Earphones lay on top. A cryptic code book lay wedged in the crevice of the desk, and beneath the desk sat an emergency power system. It looked much like a wireless model of war vintage, like the type carried in rucksacks onto the battlefields of Europe.

On closer scrutiny, Sydney decided it was more sophisticated. She could see at a glance that the whole system could be rolled back into a boxlike alcove in the desk and the louvered doors locked over it. Secrecy. Security.

Antennas protruded from the top of the communication system. She followed the thin wire to the murky window and pressed her face against the pane. The wire extended to the roof. Once she and Keeley were saddled and riding, she would look back to see whether outdoor antennas were attached to the stables. If so, this was a radio set capable of sending and receiving messages for thousands of miles. An amateur radio operator used codes that untrained listeners would never understand.

Sydney knew that Mrs. Quigley tolerated Lucas Sullivan because he had no family and few friends. She always excused him, saying, "He is committed to the care of the Admiral." But there had never been a word about Lucas's electronic skills. Now questions lurked at the back of Sydney's mind. What had lured the man to give up a full pension and medical benefits to care for one retired Admiral? Wasn't the hamlet of Stow-on-the-Woodland a quiet, sleepy village? Yet Lucas had said he sat up late at night—a perfect time to be sending messages. But where? To whom?

She glanced around for signs of a second occupant. Lucas's quarters could only serve one person. If a terrorist was harbored somewhere in the village, he wasn't hiding here in the stables.

Keeley watched her intently. "Do you like Lucas's radio?"

"Yes, but he won't like my being here and seeing it."

"I won't tell him."

Sydney felt both pleased and sad for the child. How many times had her father pledged her to silence? Young as she was, she already knew how to keep silent. Suddenly alarmed, she tilted Keeley's chin toward her. "Has Lucas—did Lucas ever touch you?"

A frown knit between the child's thin brows, a look of bewilderment. "He doesn't like children. He only lets me in his room to tell me about my papa."

"Has Danny come here with you?"

"Once. But he doesn't like the rickety stairs."

Sydney didn't either. She wondered whether he kept the stairs in disrepair to warn him of someone approaching.

"Did Gregor ever come up here?"

Her frown deepened. "Lucas doesn't like Gregor."

Sydney could understand. Gregor would not miss the contents of this room and would report back his findings to Jonas or Mrs. Quigley. No, Lucas would not trust the boy.

As they prepared to leave the room, Keeley took her hand and led her to another built-in closet. She pouted at the stubborn door, but Sydney reached up and unbolted the lock.

"See," Keeley said. "Lucas likes guns."

Sydney's spine tingled as she looked at a row of rifles. Three pistols hung on hooks above them. On one shelf lay boxes of ammunition. "You must never touch these, Keeley. Promise me?"

Before Keeley could promise, they heard Lucas's truck gunning up the driveway and squealing to a stop outside the stables. She had only seconds to wonder whether he had any radio equipment installed in his old truck and felt certain that he did. She grabbed Keeley's hand and fled down the wobbly steps. They were inside the pony's stall when Lucas found them.

He glared suspiciously at Sydney. "What are you doing?"

"We're going riding."

"Did you forget your riding stick, Miss Barrington?"

She shivered. She had left it in his room.

"Here, let me help you, Miss Barrington. You can't put the saddle on with trembling hands."

His smile was little more than a sneer as he helped her onto the saddle. He handed her the reins and went at once to lift Keeley on the pony. He was surprisingly gentle with her, a mask of incongruity. He led Keeley's pony out of the yard.

As they rode off, Sydney was afraid to glance back at the antenna wires. Cirrus clouds hovered high above them like a wispy ribbon of rainbows. The joy of the ride was gone. Sydney still felt Lucas's cold gaze on them. His trips to London took on new meaning, new possibilities. She felt convinced that he was contacting someone besides the pharmacist at the Navy exchange. But what was worse, once Lucas reached his apartment he would find Sydney's riding stick.

He would know she had been in his room.

Twenty

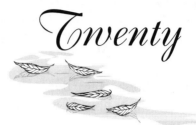

Jonas stood on the rain-drenched slope behind the manor and allowed his eyes to look over what was once a bottom story. In the early decades, his forefathers had built servants' quarters right into the hillside; and, if memory served him right, a tunnel lay beneath the stables and the main house, passing just to the left of the water tower. Jonas had searched the stables, but unless he mucked out every stall, he could not be certain that such an opening still existed.

In those early days—if he were to believe the ramblings of his father—the staff had been housed down here along with a secret gun gallery that hid the weaponry from the Cornwall forces. Then a hundred years ago, a flood almost washed the village away, and eventually those rooms had been cemented off.

Now tangled vines climbed the back walls and prickly brambles covered what had once been windows. Try as he did, he could not remember where the back entry had been. He often explored this area as a boy; now it looked hopeless.

Somewhere behind that cement there was a perfect hiding area for a man on the run, but only if he had someone supplying him sustenance. Boris was too loyal a Brit to hide anyone and too unsteady on his feet to wander behind the manor on this uneven, slippery ground. Nor was it likely that Griselda would join forces with anyone to befriend Conon O'Reilly. She would care for his children, but there she would draw the line.

But what if Conon remembered that a refuge lay beneath the manor? Conon would be clever enough to find it. Whichever way Jonas's search led, he risked betraying someone, and it kept boiling down to three people: Danny and Keeley O'Reilly and Abigail. One thing was certain. There were ample rooms in the manor to hide a dozen men. He had covered every inch of paneling on the second floor, and no hollow sounds indicated a space behind them. Plowing through furnished rooms on the west wing, ghostlike under their dustcovers, he found the original blueprints with proof that a bottom floor had once existed.

Jonas stepped forward in his muddy boots and began tearing at the bramble with his bare hands, searching for cracks in the masonry. He tore at the vines and trampled them with his boot. He brushed angrily at the damp strands of hair straying over his brow and kept tearing at nature's barricade. Thirty minutes later his hands were bleeding, his clothes sopping with rain and sweat.

Wiping the sweat and hair from his brow, he scanned the back of the manor once more, his gaze settling on the west wing. Lucas stood in the Admiral's window watching him. As their eyes locked, Lucas let the curtain fall in place.

Jonas's hands stung as he walked around the manor and came face-to-face with Sydney on the front steps.

"You're hurt," she said.

"Just a few scratches."

She took his hands in hers and turned them palms up. "Those are more than scratches, Jonas. What have you been doing?"

"I was trying to break through some bramble."

"Without your gardening tools? Come inside and I'll wash those wounds for you."

She led him into Abigail's room, past the sleeping woman and straight into the washroom. He winced as she scrubbed the wounds and poured antibiotics on the deepest cuts. In spite of the stinging pain, he could not take his eyes from her face.

"You've been gone the last two days," Sydney said.

"So have you."

"I flew to Germany to visit our associate plant there, and then I went back up to the shipyard."

"What a busy woman you are."

She smiled. "I'm getting everything ready in case we win those carrier bids. Where were you?"

"I was on business too. Griselda probably thought we stole away together. She's a romantic at heart, you know."

Sydney felt a crimson flush on her cheeks. "So, where were you, Jonas?"

"I drove into Northwood to meet with my commanding officer, but he was called away unexpectedly. So I checked some files."

"Files on your Irish terrorist?"

"You know things like that are classified."

"At least off limits to me?"

"Jonas!" Abigail called, stirring from her sleep. "I forgot. Gregor said you have company at the cottage. The gentleman is waiting for you."

He held up his bandaged hands. "Thanks, Sydney."

Sydney sighed as he left.

"Missing him already?" Abigail asked.

Sydney propped herself on the edge of Abigail's bed. "I definitely missed him while I was gone. I thought things would be different when I came back, but I still feel as though his dead fiancée keeps coming between us. Abigail, why did she go to Ireland alone?"

Abigail squeezed her hand. "A woman in love does foolish things. Their wedding was delayed. Their honeymoon canceled. Rather than face her friends, Louise took the trip alone."

"What was she like?"

"Are you asking me whether she was anything like you?"

"I guess I am."

"You're two completely different people, but both lovely. To answer your question though, Louise was sweet-tempered, sweet-scented as a bouquet of roses, as fresh and pure as the Windrush. And shy. She was six years younger than Jonas, but it wasn't just the age. It was Louise. She grew up in the shelter of the parish, living under the pressure of being the daughter of the Bishop of Monkton. With Jonas she experienced a new sense of freedom—a stretching of her personality."

"Were they happy?"

"They were in love. I don't know if they were happy—that's something different. She never adjusted to Jonas being gone so many months at a time. I think she wanted him to give up the Service and settle down in Stow-on-the-Woodland."

I would never ask him to do that, Sydney thought. *Give up his dream. Give up his career.*

"And she was afraid of his flying. She never flew herself."

"Did you like her?"

"Most assuredly. Perhaps because she was so in love with Jonas. So transparent. Totally honest. And yet sometimes she wasn't honest about what she really wanted. They were refurbishing the east wing for their own quarters—"

"No wonder he was shocked when Mrs. Quigley put me in the east wing. And why he fussed even more when we moved you down beside me. If Griselda had only said something."

"I think she did it deliberately—so Jonas would let go of memories. But once when Louise was decorating the east wing, I found her hanging up new curtains and crying. She wanted a cottage of their own. Just a small place. No extra rooms. Just a place for the two of them."

"But there would have been children."

"Childbirth frightened her. Her own mother died when Louise was born. I don't think there would have been children."

"How sad. Watching Jonas with Gregor, I think he would make a wonderful father."

207

Abigail's mouth curved into another smile. "Jonas doesn't see himself as a family man. But there are so many positive things about him. He's a skilled pilot, an excellent horseman, an avid sportsman. He helps take care of Sir James and tends the sheep and works in the garden."

"I don't hear him complain."

"No, bless his heart, he does what he does without rancor, but he must be longing for the day when he can return to his Navy commission on board ship. I pray for that return. I have prayed for all my children. For you too. But mostly I prayed for Jonas, even before his birth. I'm so proud of him." From her window, they watched Jonas and Gregor pushing through the gate, Jonas towering above the boy. "Right this moment seeing those two, I have everything to live for—and I have everything to die for."

To Sydney's startled frown, she said, "Don't look so worried, dear child. I am not afraid of dying, for when this old heart of mine gives out for the last time, I will simply leave the Cotswolds and be in heaven. I've roamed these hills since childhood. I can't think of any place more beautiful, yet heaven will be more glorious. I will have a new heart. A new body. One of the first things I'm going to ask is, 'Dear Lord, why did you forgive me so much? Why did you love me so much?'"

Her voice grew unsteady. "There's a poem of someone asking that question of Jesus. He answered by stretching out His arms as He died on the cross."

"Abigail, I could never believe the way you do. I've messed up so much of my life."

She chuckled. "Oh, my dear child, no one could have marred the clay more than I did. Think about it. One day soon I think you will understand what I am saying about God and forgiveness."

"You sound like Reverend Rainford-Simms."

"He's the one who taught me the extent of forgiveness."

"I think Jonas feels the same way, but he seldom says anything."

"He's carrying bitterness against the IRA. When he lets that go, God will heal him. Maybe if he went to Ireland and saw the place where Louise died, then he could put it all to rest."

"Have you told him that, Abigail?"

"No, that's between himself and his God."

"Does it worry you that he will go back to sea soon?"

"I try not to think about it. But sometimes I think Jonas is itching for an act of war that will thrust him back to sea duty—and free him from the responsibility of everything here. More action in the Gulf or anywhere that would lead him to another promotion and eventually to the Admiralty."

"He has such big dreams."

"No, only one. To finally attain his father's approval."

"Abigail, I find his father charming."

"Most women do. But as a father, he's not a very warm man. The Admiral's wife on the other hand was sophisticated and gracious. They rather went their separate ways. She loved the Cotswolds. James loved the city. So she brought their London friends to the manor for glorious parties and dances."

She reflected for a moment. "The parties ended when she died out on the wolds while horseback riding. Soon after the accident I took the train to Gordonstoun to tell Jonas. I think he knew when he saw me. I opened my arms, and he just flew into them."

"Have you always been close?"

"Lately he's been avoiding me. But he's always in my heart. I've loved him for a thousand reasons."

"Special to you?"

"More than special. But you asked me about Louise. I must tell you she was delightful, but no more so than you. You're more guarded with your affections. Less sure of yourself that way. With Louise, there was never any question about how she felt about Jonas."

"I feel uneasy around him—as though we are always a party of three. Louise comes silently between us."

Abigail smiled sympathetically. "I think what you see as uneasiness, Jonas sees as self-assurance, independence. The other day he told me that he might end up sailing on a ship that you built. Louise didn't have your confidence or your business strengths. Nor your sophistication. But she was lovely. Dear to all of us. And so terribly young to die that way."

Keeley burst into the room and flung herself at Sydney. "I looked everywhere for you!"

"I've been right here with Abigail."

"Gregor said you were with Jonas."

Abigail touched the child's hand. "I see you've brought a book with you. Would you let me read it to you?"

"You never read to me before, Miss Abigail."

"I was sick right after you came."

"Did I make you sick?"

"No, dear child." She patted the bed. "Climb up here with me, and I'll read to you."

"Read, Abigail," Keeley cried impatiently as she settled against the pillows. Abigail opened the book and flattened the first page. By the time they reached the last page, Keeley had fallen asleep.

"Well, I've lost my touch," Abigail said. "Sydney, when I saw how quickly you took to Keeley, I prayed that you would take up my work. But I won't thrust my burden on your shoulders. There comes a time when we must finish our own course—when the work is complete. And there must come a time when *you* follow your own heart."

"Are you talking about Keeley or Jonas now?"

Their eyes met across the sleeping child. "Both."

"Abigail, were you never in love?"

She laughed. "Many times. But only twice with all my heart. Once when I was young—and once when I was foolish."

"Did neither man want to work with you and the children?"

210

She answered in riddles. "One did. It was forced on the other one." Abigail tucked her blanket around the sleeping child and settled more comfortably against her pillows. "You know Santos Garibaldi now. I wish you could meet his father. Remember, I told you Victor and I met on the beaches of Dunkirk."

"Then you *were* in love with him?"

"No, but in true Italian fashion he thought himself in love with me. Our friendship began when Victor found me weeping along the roadside during the evacuation of Dunkirk. You'd have to know him to know how sweet he was. Even with the Germans swooping overhead, Victor promised that we would both reach safety."

Her voice softened, saddened, as she retreated into the past. "It was the spring of 1940. Czechoslovakia and Poland had already surrendered, and the German scout cars were speeding toward the Luxembourg frontier. Vice Admiral Ramsay sat in his command post in Dover, and what was left of the British Expeditionary Forces were fleeing toward Dunkirk, hoping, praying that there would be ships there to rescue them. Nine days of deliverance for some, captivity for others, death for the unfortunate." Abigail's voice became softer still.

"The sea was littered with mines and the shattered remains of rescue boats. Vessels of every size zigzagged across the English Channel in the darkness, some colliding with the mines." Her fingers plucked nervously at a stray thread. "I have tried to forget the bodies in the water and the dead along the road to Dunkirk. But I will always remember Victor Garibaldi and Neil Irwin, because I owe my life to them.

"In spite of the darkness looming over the continent, I had insisted on going to Belgium to visit a school friend. Now we were stumbling along the road with thousands of civilians fleeing toward the coast, the younger pushing the elderly and injured in wheelbarrows. The burning city and the harbor lay ahead.

"An hour into the march, I lost sight of my friend when we dove for cover. When the sound of the planes faded at last, I climbed from the ditch. 'Gabrielle. Gabrielle!' I called.

"My friend never answered. Smoke curled from the cart in front of me. Slowly the living began to stand. There was no time for weeping for the dead; all of us fell into line and moved toward the burning city.

Sydney touched Abigail's trembling hand. "Abigail, I didn't mean to bring back so much pain. You don't have to go on."

"It's all right, child. That road to Dunkirk lives in my memory." Her smile grew faint. "Strange as it may seem, Sydney, Dunkirk led to my life's work, for it was after the third Luftwaffe attack that I saw two small children standing against a fence, crying. When I pushed my way to them, they cried out in German and I recoiled. They were the enemy. The older boy's lip trembled. He was as afraid of me as I was of him. '*Mutter? Vater?*' I asked, unable to touch them. He shook his head and pointed to a woman lying motionless face down a few yards from us.

"I forced myself to read the name tags pinned to the boys' tattered sweaters. Hermann. And Isaac—the younger one with the dirt-smudged face and cavernous eyes. I knew by their names that they were the hated Jewish children. The German army must not overtake them. There would be no mercy. I held out my hands. They took them, and without looking back at their dead mother, went with me through the deserted towns of Flanders, stepping around broken windows, tripping over suitcases with broken straps, and worse, climbing over lifeless bodies. Somewhere along the way, we came across another dead German soldier whose belt buckle read: *God is with us.*

"I almost gave up then. Where was God in all of this? With the enemy? I lay down with the children and wept. Victor Garibaldi found us there. In broken English, he said soothingly, 'I will protect you and your sons. So young. All of you so young.'

"He was young himself and handsome. An artist, I would learn later, a young man fleeing from the fascist regime in his own country. 'No family. You will be my family now,' he said as he tapped his chest. 'Twenty. I am a man.'

"I held tightly to the boys. As our world exploded around us, Victor, Hermann, Isaac, and I pushed along in the throng like a family of four. We were just one more family of evacuees fleeing toward the burning city of Dunkirk. Then the rumors reached us. Only British soldiers would be evacuated. Everyone else would be turned away—even the French and Belgians who had fought beside them.

"That's when we met Neil Irwin, a bewhiskered British Tommy with sun-blond hair who had not lost spirit and who was hurrying his unit along. But the strafing kept on, and some of the men in his unit died. 'There's no point in going on,' I told him. 'We'll die before we get there. And they're not evacuating civilians.'

"'You'll never know until we get there, mate' he told me. 'But if it's just soldiers, then we'll make soldiers out of you and your husband. Get yourselves kitted up.' He clamped his jaw as he stripped the uniforms from two of his dead comrades and handed them to Victor and me. 'Quick,' he commanded us.

"As he shoved the steel helmet on my head, it slipped down over my ears. The Lee-Enfield rifle was too heavy for me to carry and the khaki greatcoat swept my ankles, but I managed a faint smile for his efforts. I asked him what we should do about the children. With gunfire exploding behind us, he winked and put khaki undershirts and sweaters on the boys. 'We'll find a way, mate,' he assured me."

Abigail paused for a moment, then went on. "When we reached the port, it was true. They were only evacuating British soldiers. Everyone else was being turned back. Pushed aside. I put my finger to my lips to silence the children. One word in German and there would be no mercy. Victor begged the soldiers passing by in canvas-covered trucks to let us ride, but angry men shoved us away. In despair, he said, 'But these are children. And this woman—she is British.'

"They turned a deaf ear, but not Neil. He looked at the mass of troops standing silently on the sands, waiting their turn for evacuation. 'I'm not leaving unless you go with me, Abigail,' he said.

"He boosted Hermann to his shoulders and ordered Victor to carry Isaac. With the determination of a man bent on living and taking his friends with him, Neil led us over the bloody beaches of Dunkirk to the water's edge.

"A dinghy was loading, ready to carry more evacuees back to the waiting ships. 'Soldiers only,' the helmsman said.

"Neil took a firm grip on the man's arm. 'If you want to get back to your vessel, take this family on board. Or I will keep you here with me and you can wait it out with my men, but this family goes.' Within twenty minutes we reached a pleasure yacht, part of Admiral Ramsay's cockleshell navy. 'Sir,' the helmsman said, 'I told them we're not to take women and children.'

"'This is my ship, Smithers,' the captain said, smiling at me. 'And I'm not a man to leave a woman and children stranded. Bring them on board.'

Abigail brushed a tear from her eye. "Neil lifted Hermann into the captain's arms. Then he held out his hand to me, smiling as he shielded me from the whistling crash of the German shells. 'Don't worry, my love. I'll catch the next vessel,' he said."

She wiped her dry lips. "I was sick all the way across the channel but so grateful to reach Dover safely. We were greeted by volunteers passing out strong tea and sandwiches and meat pies. We were treated like royalty and then one of the volunteers told me that Admiral Bertram Ramsay had been informed that a ship of odds and sods had come ashore with a woman and two Jewish children and an Italian artist.

"She quoted the Admiral as saying, 'That's bloody marvelous. Sounds like a nice family.'

"'Should we send them back, sir?'" the helmsman asked. 'The food is intended for the soldiers.'

"But the volunteer told me that Admiral Ramsay lowered his field glasses. 'Let them come ashore. No soldier who reached the safety of English soil will turn that family away. There will be plenty of apples and sweet biscuits and chocolate for the children. And have the women rally up some warm clothing and blankets for the children. This is England, young man. Welcome them.'"

Abigail's voice choked with emotion. "It was days before I saw Neil Irwin again. But he was my first love. We fell in love quickly and were engaged shortly after Dunkirk, but my family wanted me to wait until after the war to marry him. And there were the children—I had nowhere to send them. After a short rest, Neil went back to battle—as a British Commando. Before he left he put his helmet on my head again and said, 'Well, mate. We'll have to wait until after the war to keep your parents happy. But never forget, Abigail, how much I love you.'"

Her eyes grew misty. "I waited for him to come back all through the war."

"But you never married him?"

"No, he was killed in Normandy. After that it just seemed like I was meant to go on mothering the hidden children of wars. I loved Neil and I've always thought he would have wanted me to go on taking care of children."

"Abigail, you mentioned two loves. What about the *foolish* one?"

"Another time, child. Perhaps we can talk about it then." She placed her hand on Sydney's. "But follow your heart, Sydney, as I did with Neil, and you will have no regrets."

Twenty-one

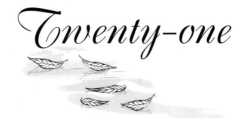

Jonas found Captain McIntyre waiting for him in front of the cottage. He wore his full dress uniform, making no secret of his presence in the village.

"I've just come from seeing your father, Willoughby."

"Then you know the state of his health?"

"I know he is a man still to be admired. He was commanding his ship right there in the west wing. We talked about the Falklands. He remembered everything clearly."

"It's only the present that's lost, sir. Dad spends most of his time in the past, standing on an imaginary bridge giving orders. He rarely takes an interest in the *Navy News* anymore."

He took the captain inside. "Tea? Biscuits?"

The Admiral's steward served tea. "Commander, your father is not happy with you on board here. He tells me you gave up your future with the Navy when you turned down the minesweeper. You didn't change your career course with your father's approval."

"That's something I've never had."

The captain let it pass. "Perhaps your father is more aware of what's going on around him than any of us know."

"He's more lucid since Dr. Wallis took him off narcotics. The only thing he's on now is heart meds. But he doesn't have much of a life anymore."

"I take it you're still angry with the Navy for retiring your father?"

"You put him down like an old ship. Even the *HMS Cavalier* fared better. At least they attempted to salvage the *Cavalier* from the scrap pile. My dad gave his best to the Navy too."

"The final duty is never easy, Commander."

Now that the steam was blowing, he couldn't stop it. "I still say the ship ended up with more recognition and a permanent berth. What did my father get for his long career?"

The captain snapped off his answer. "Your dad was knighted by the Queen. He had every honor a man could earn. He had a long career. An excellent service record. And he had 250 acres to come home to; Broadshire Manor is no small final docking."

Jonas glanced out the window where the sheep grazed. "But you put Dad out to pasture long before he planned to retire."

"Commander, there's something you don't know. Toward the end of his career, he failed to keep appointments that were on his schedule. He rambled when he gave reports. He was found wandering at the wrong tube station carrying high priority briefs."

Stunned, Jonas asked, "Why wasn't I notified?"

"The Admiral's doing. You were not to know. Nothing was to interrupt your career. That was the Admiral's stipulation. He'd go quietly with that promise. The Admiral was one of the most respected men in the Service. He was no quitter. He went out with his head high. In full uniform. I can still see him walking away and getting into the car provided for him. He never looked back."

Jonas ran his hands through his hair. "I don't know what to say. I suppose I did disappoint him by not taking that promotion."

"With your fine record, something else will come along." He turned to the business at hand. "Did you take the Admiral's steward into your confidence?"

Jonas's stomach took a dive. "I'm afraid so, sir. I tried to enlist his help in finding O'Reilly, but Lucas told me not to dirty up Stow-on-the-Woodland with Navy rumors."

"Be careful whom you trust. I know Lucas Sullivan has been with the Admiral for twenty years, but without polishing the Admiral's boots, he might not have made it in this man's Navy." He rested his elbows on the arms of the chair. "Tell me, how is your assignment going, Commander? Give an accounting."

Jonas knew better than McIntyre how little he had accomplished. "I spend most of my evenings at Chutman's Pub meeting old neighbors, being introduced to new ones. They all have legitimate reasons for living in Stow-on-the-Woodland."

Jonas knew everybody in the hamlet by name. He knew which men found employment out of the village and which ones played darts left-handed down at Chutman's. He could name the men who had searched the woods and combed the riverbank the night of the shooting. Many had strong opinions about the negotiations on the Northern Ireland conflict; none had an Irish connection strong enough to want the conflict to go on. And none of them cared whether the Irishman was found or not.

"So you haven't accomplished anything except to improve your dart game at the pub? I don't believe that for a minute, Willoughby. Have you checked out the women who live here too?"

That was a stab in the dark at Abigail Broderick again. "I did locate the O'Reilly children. Here at the manor."

Not a muscle twitched in the captain's face. "And you're just now reporting that to me? So where is Conon O'Reilly?"

"The men here stand to a man that Conon left the village alive. As far as they're concerned now, Stow-on-the-Woodland is a long way from Ireland. I've known most of these men all my life. I can't believe any of them is aligned with the IRA movement."

"Or you refuse to believe it? We'll take the children in."

"Captain, that will create a disturbance we don't want. Their father left them on the doorstep the night Abigail Broderick had her heart attack. Abigail is highly respected in this village for her work with the children and her fairness with others. The entire village would rally if you tried to take the children." He hesitated. "Abigail is getting better each day. Sooner or later, she will tell me where Conon is, if she knows."

McIntyre stood and squared his cap. "We've taken the peace agreements as far as we can, Willoughby. The only thing standing in the way of a permanent peace would be the IRA factional groups still holding out. Even Sinn Fein can't tell us where they are, but men like O'Reilly could ruin it for all of us. I trust that your loyalty to Miss Broderick is not standing in your way?"

"Politics have never been important to her. Conon came here just to bring his children to her. His boyhood memories are here in the village, but not his Irish ties."

McIntyre leaned forward. "Don't be too sure. Conon is not a man to work alone. I have to give him credit. He wanted his children safe and took a risk coming here. You're not close to airports or train depots. But O'Reilly must have had help coming in—and he needs help going out."

"So he's locked in, Commander. And so am I."

Jonas stood, his palms together, his forefingers to his lips. As he processed the last few days, he knew he was fighting for his career and his reputation.

"We were friends once until we disagreed politically. But I can't ignore his children, sir. I understand where Abigail was coming from when she took them in. But keep in mind, she sent Conon away. Whether she knows where he is now, I don't know."

He glanced up and found Captain McIntyre watching him sympathetically. "The Admiral told me there's a lovely young American staying here at the manor. The Admiral was never one to miss a beautiful woman. He said quite lucidly that it's a shame for you to find someone again and not be able to make a commitment to her. Tell me, how does she feel about O'Reilly?"

"She thinks of him as the father of Keeley and Danny."

"And she is influencing you?"

"She calls it a cat-and-mouse game. She suggested that the village is a perfect place for an IRA encampment."

"She's right. They could blend right in with this community while planning for the future. Whether you believe it or not, Willoughby, they may have been here for months or even years. When the time comes, violence could erupt again."

"Then finding Conon becomes secondary, sir."

"Explain yourself, Commander."

"Those who are sheltering him become more important. If he is hiding somewhere here in Stow-on-the-Woodland, I'd be forced to look at the men in this household and find excuses for them. As it is, I look at the schoolmaster—a single man who travels a lot and is an expert shot—and I think, are you the one protecting Conon? I challenge the Irish owner of Chutman's Pub to a game of darts and find myself drawing a web around him, wondering whether he was planted here. He's lived here for twenty years and I no longer trust him. Last night I awakened in a sweat accusing Rainford-Simms of Irish connections. Do you know who he is, Captain?"

"The name sounds familiar."

"He's the rector. He would have been my father-in-law."

"And I've put you in the middle, scrutinizing your friends."

"You've put me to the test, sir. Whoever it is—whoever took Conon in—I will find it difficult to end an old friendship."

The captain shook Jonas's hand warmly. "I'm flying back to Belfast for another go at the conference table. The end is definitely in sight. But if you need me, call me on the red-alert line. Someone on my staff will plug you through without delay."

Jeff VanBurien walked into the tiny kitchen in the vicarage and startled Kersten. The tray in her hand crashed to the floor, the tea and a soft-boiled egg curling together on the tray.

"Are you eating in your room?" he asked as he bent to help her clean up the mess.

"Don't ask."

He touched her wrist. "Kersten, I know from watching that this isn't the life you want. Why don't you think about going back to Maine and getting a job? If you're unhappy there, I'll help you find employment in Chicago."

"Even if they needed artists in the Windy City, I couldn't leave the reverend. Not right now."

"I've seen you out on the hills painting. May I come and watch the next time?"

"If you want." She sniffed as they stood. "Jeff, I'm an awful cook. I hope I'm a better artist."

"Who was the tray for, Kersten? Chan and I get our own breakfast, and Reverend Rainford-Simms can't be ill. I saw him out walking in his garden a few moments ago."

"He prays out there or something."

"Is he praying away some kind of trouble?"

"Please, Jeff. Don't ask. He's a good man."

"I think he could be breaking the laws of the land—especially if there's another guest staying in this house."

Kersten's chin jutted forward stoutly. "I know he's troubled about what's happening, but he feels it's his duty as a man of the church to deal kindly with everyone who comes to him."

She thinks I know more than I do. "When are you going to paint again?" he asked.

"This afternoon if I can get away."

"I'll do up the dishes for you. Will that help?"

Her tears spilled over. "Can you boil eggs too?"

He laughed. "For you, yes. Here, take my handkerchief. I can't stomach a woman crying."

She grabbed the linen cloth and blew lustily. "Now go, please, before the reverend comes in and finds me crying."

He left her and went straight to his room and closed the door. "Chandler, we have a bigger problem than Edmund Gallagher. We can settle that one legally. But I think the rumors about an Irish terrorist are real. I think he's holed up in this parish."

Chan gave an amused wave of his hand. "Well, he's not in any of the shops or the pub or in those cottages nearby."

"So you have been thinking about it too? The missing man can only be in one of two places big enough to hide him. That manor where Sydney is staying—or here in the old rectory."

"You're dead serious, big brother?"

"Quite serious. Have you pawed through the trash lately?"

"I don't make a habit of it."

"You should. Kersten has been carrying out trash bags filled with bloody bandages. Take my word for it, Chan. We'll have to wait a couple of days for a good look around in the vicarage when Charles is gone and Kersten is out as well."

"Charles will be at the church for at least an hour and a half on Sunday. That's when Kersten escapes to the hills to paint so she doesn't have to go to the service."

"We'll check this place out on Sunday. One of us better go to church. Chan, you're more into this God business than I am."

Chan studied his brother. "Sunday it is then. But I doubt you'll find anything. Charles isn't going to break the law."

"We'll know more on Sunday."

Behind the secret Jacobean wall in a windowless room, a weakened Conon O'Reilly lay on his narrow cot with his sweaty face close to the panel. He smothered his cough until

"Gallagher is holding something over his head. A breach of confidentiality is my guess. I told Wallis I have no legal claims in this country, but if he's honest with me, I think I can help him. But that's not what I wanted to talk to you about. I'm on to something different this morning. The harboring of a terrorist here in Stow-on-the-Woodland is no longer a joke to me."

She started to tell Jeff about Lucas's radio system. But accuse him falsely? No, she would wait until she was certain.

"I gave the rectory a once-over, but the whole property needs a more thorough search, including that domed-roof dovecote," Jeff said.

"It's boarded off."

"Then tear those boards down when Chan and I drive Charles into London for his meeting with the Archbishop of Canterbury."

"The senior cleric? Is Charles in trouble with the Church of England?"

"He doesn't say. If they wanted to retire him, they'd do so. If he harbored an Irish fugitive, then he's heading to Lambeth Palace for a dressing-down. It's up to you and Jonas to check this place out while we're gone. Chan plans to see his wife, and I made an appointment with the senior member at Gallagher's firm."

"You're going to talk to them about Edmund?"

"They can't conduct a reputable firm with a dishonest lawyer on their staff. Blackmailing Wallis or destroying Broderick are no more acceptable here than in our own country. I'll be careful. And I'll be back to keep a watch on you a few more days."

"So what do you have in mind for me to do?"

"It regards Charles. I have to admit I'm not always certain that Charles is with the whole program. But down at the pub, Chan and Jonas take offense if anyone calls him dotty. At least he's smart enough to know what's going on. That's where you come in."

he was certain the Americans had left their room. Shortly, Kersten or Lucas would come to redress his festering wounds. He must remember to warn them to destroy the old dressings at once. He had no desire to put harm in the reverend's path. The man had been good to him. Kind, benevolent.

Conon longed to be gone by Sunday, but the Americans had no way of finding him here. He was safe in this airless room that smelled of his own rotting body. How many of his IRA comrades had died in even less favorable conditions? With great effort, he turned on his back. The motion increased the throbbing in his gut. Lucas had assured him there were four men in the village waiting to take up arms when the time came, the schoolmaster for one. Other strong men were in close proximity. But in Conon's confusion, he tried to define the loyalty of the schoolmaster, so convinced was he that the schoolmaster had shot him.

Conon coughed again and winced from the pain. *Will I ever be well again?* he wondered.

Could Lucas really get him out of here alive? Or had his usefulness run its full course? He wished the priest would come in for his daily visit. Priest? No, he had that wrong. That was from his boyhood. The vicar was Protestant. But he wore a white clerical collar as the priests back home had done, and he carried a prayer book when he came. Charles was a mild-mannered man, ducking low to enter the Jacobean room. He had strange beliefs and firm convictions. He'd sit on the only chair available and visit. Never condemning. Always insisting before he left to open that little book and read its comforting words.

Conon tried to tell him that there was a place in hell—if hell existed—for men like himself. Yesterday Conon tried to convey to Reverend Rainford-Simms that it was too late. That his soul was already condemned to eternal damnation.

Charles had stood, a very tall man towering above Conon's cot, an old man with gentle eyes. "Son, there's still time," he had said.

Conon closed his eyes and drifted into an empty void, then fought for consciousness again. He ached to go outside and breathe in the fresh air. Longed to stand facing the golden hills that he had loved as a boy and glance up at the manor where he had once lived. Tonight when the Americans and the cleric slept, he could inch his way outside and crawl on his hands and knees back to the manor. Keeley. Danny. Rorie. No, Rorie was dead. Keeley and Danny, his own flesh and blood, were still alive. He ached even to whisper their names. The dankness of the room could not blot out the sweetness of their faces. Rorie, his fiery redhead. Danny, the image of Rorie. Keeley, too much like himself.

Danny. Keeley. You are safe, he thought. *Safe with Abigail.*

He drifted, and this time he could not rally himself but fell into a deep slumber that numbed his mind and took away the pain, the fear of dying—at least for a little while.

On Sunday Sydney walked up the narrow aisle of St. Michael's while the church bell was ringing and squeezed into one of the hard pews, two rows behind Jonas. As the organ played, she studied the stony interior with its tall pillars and high vaulted ceiling. The sun poured through the stained-glass windows. The names of the Archbishops of Canterbury were etched in marble on the back wall, the life of Christ recorded in the windows.

The songs and message were unfamiliar. She kept her eyes on the back of Jonas's head and wondered if he understood what Charles was saying. Her thoughts wandered again, her eyes straying to the window behind Reverend Rainford-Simms. Was it possible that she was the lamb that Christ was carrying?

As the sermon ended, she focused on the white baptismal font that stood to her right. She tried to visualize Lady Willoughby with Jonas in her arms and the Admiral in full uniform—proud man—standing beside her. Neither approving nor disapproving. Simply lending his powerful image. And

Abigail—where was she when the bishop touched Jonas and said, "In the name of the Father and Son and Holy Ghost"?

The service was over. Jonas slipped out of the church and strode briskly toward the manor. Had he seen her? How could he miss her in such a small congregation? Saddened by his rejection, she made her way to the vicarage where Jeff waited for her.

"Good morning, Miss Sunshine. Was the sermon that bad?"

"If you had been there you could judge for yourself."

He tilted her chin up and looked down into her eyes. "You were there for both of us. But I hope you didn't attend just because Jonas Willoughby was going to be there. I see what's happening—and you're only going to get hurt."

"Am I that obvious?"

"Only to another man who fancies himself in love with you. Don't get me wrong. I like Jonas. But he has an ongoing love affair with the Royal Navy. In the old days they were discouraged from thinking about marriage until after they were thirty. That's obstacle enough, but Jonas is still picking up the pieces from his fiancée's death. Chan and I don't want you hurt."

She straightened her shoulders. "Why aren't you off with the young artist? She's pretty enough to take your fancy."

"She does. And she's in trouble enough to need my help. But I had something else to do while Charles was otherwise engaged."

"You didn't confront Edmund Gallagher?"

"I can't get past a phone call with him. He's probably digging into his law books to come up with answers for us. Just don't make any appointments with him, Syd. We'll keep Gallagher guessing that way. I've called Gallagher's London firm. I don't think they will like what he is doing to the doctor in town."

"Marshall Wallis? He's a good man. He's guarded around me but kind to his patients. Abigail adores him."

He leaned forward and lowered his voice and mapped out a plan, daring in its possibilities, threatening in its outcome. And it put Sydney and Jonas in the thick of the battle.

"Oh, Jeff. You can't expect me to confront Charles here at the vicarage? And Abigail? I'm not sure I can accuse them—"

"See how things go. They both trust you."

"And I'm about to break their trust."

Sydney stood on the flower-lined path between the church and the vicarage and waited for Charles. She saw him at last. He had discarded his clerical robe and was returning to the vicarage with a tiny kitten cradled against him. Charles came the rest of the way toward her tall as timber, yet his shoulders bent forward like the branch of an old oak. His wise eyes counseled her without a word; the bluish-gray threads of his Shetland sweater enhanced their silvery blue. "My dear, if I had known you were waiting for me, I would have come right home."

She murmured, "I didn't mean to intrude. Or come uninvited."

"Intrude, my child? Hardly; I keep the doors of the church open at all hours for those who come to reflect and pray."

"I didn't come to pray, Charles."

"Thinking and sorting life out are permissible here too." His eyes twinkled, and she felt comforted in his presence. Though his thick head of hair was as white as snowfall, aging him, Sydney did not find him dotty at all.

He put the kitten on the ground. "She's my most faithful parishioner. She comes every day. Of course, a saucer of milk tempts her." He smiled. "Sydney, I watched you in the service this morning. I think you are quite close to the Man of peace."

"God, you mean?"

"God's Son."

"Did you know my parents were missionaries?"

"Abigail told me. They were married here at St. Michael's—and your mother baptized here. You had a godly beginning, child."

Sydney looked into his kindly face. She had never known anyone so peaceful, and she was about to take his peace away.

He smiled again, the warm smile still ministering to her as he grasped her hand. "Now then, how can I help you?"

The direct approach was best. "Reverend, the night of the explosion down by the bridge—were the church doors open then?"

"Of course. The doors are never locked." He sighed. "They were barred shut for too many months before I came. But it wasn't an explosion that night. It was gunfire."

"If you heard gunfire, would you go to help the injured?"

"That would be my pattern." He peered intently over his rimmed glasses. "I'm an old man, but I did my fair share of stumbling in the dark that night."

"Jonas would argue that your purpose of coming to this hamlet was to light the darkness."

"So Jonas does speak of me?"

"Often. He's fond of you."

"He avoids me. Jonas is too busy for a cup of tea with an old friend. I think he's forgotten the way to the vicarage."

"He's been busy settling the affairs at the manor."

"Tell him, if he needs my help, I'm available seven days a week. But at least he found his way to the service this morning."

Sydney was running in circles, avoiding the crucial topic. "You remind Jonas of Louise." Her throat tightened at the word.

"It's his bitterness against the way she died that keeps us apart." She saw the tremor in his hand. "Louise was killed in an IRA bombing, perhaps by one man. We will never know for certain. Jonas's war is against anyone who bears allegiance to the IRA. I understand his bitterness—I struggled with it myself. But vengeance will only destroy him."

228

He had steered her from the night in question. "Do you think that terrorist was wounded the night of the shooting, Charles?"

"Such is the rumor."

"Conon O'Reilly was in town that night."

The bushy brows arched with amusement. "You've obviously been looking into matters. And you have a theory?"

"My friends and I think Conon stumbled into the church that night. Wounded, perhaps. If he did, you would never turn him out of the church. Was he here, Charles? Is he still here?"

"Conon is one of Abigail's boys. If he went anywhere, wouldn't he go to her for protection?" He pointed to the door that led into his study. "We'd better sit down and talk."

"Only if you're honest with me."

Again the bushy brows arched. "If I am a man who lights the darkness, as you say, then I must be honest."

He turned abruptly, walked into the room, and went to his model train. He seemed distracted as though he had forgotten that she had followed him inside.

"Charles, the Windrush flows behind the church, doesn't it?"

His shoulders stiffened. "You seem to know for certain. But it's only a small stream that branches off there."

"Yesterday, the children and I were out walking. Gregor ran ahead of us as he always does. He's the one who found the trail that leads from the water up to the brow of the hill where the church stands. I think Conon could have reached the church that way after he was shot trying to leave Miss Broderick's."

He turned. For the first time, there was coolness in his eyes. "Miss Broderick is not a violent woman."

"No. I didn't mean that. Someone else shot him. But I think he found refuge with you."

"Could one terrorist outwit all the men in this village?"

"He was that kind of man, Reverend. He's been on the run since Omagh. His little children miss him."

"Such a long time to keep running," he reflected. "And you really think I am harboring a fugitive?"

"You spoke on the prodigal coming home this morning. To you, Conon would seem like a prodigal coming home. Home to Abigail. Home to the manor. Home to the village."

"Home to the church. To the Shepherd," he said.

"You're the only one in the village that no one suspects."

"But you suspect me? It would be quite difficult for me to harbor a fugitive with Jeff and Chandler staying with me."

"If not in the vicarage, then perhaps in the church? Or in that old roundabout dovecote out behind the parish?"

He flipped the switch. The train chugged along the track, its whistle blowing. "Why would I protect someone when my daughter was killed in an IRA bombing? She was the child of my old age. The delight of my life."

"You are one of the few people who would find the strength to do so. Or maybe you did it to protect Jonas from himself."

"Louise went on that trip to Ireland with my blessing. I sent her to her death. We don't know why she strayed into that thickly wooded valley. There was concern at first—because she was engaged to a naval officer. . . . The terrorists never gave my daughter a chance. She was just in the wrong place at the wrong time. . . . But if she had to die, it was good that she died there. She loved Ireland. Loved the people."

Your thoughts aren't scattered, she thought. *You have your wits about you.*

"Charles, you still haven't answered me. Are you hiding Conon O'Reilly in your home or in the church?"

"If I did something like that, may God forgive me." He smiled wearily. "I'm tired, Sydney. I must go and rest now."

Twenty-two

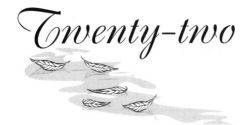

Sydney's global ambitions as a young executive slipped into second gear as her call with Randolph Iverson ended. These days her waking hours were peppered with thoughts of a British pilot and a motherless child. She dared not mention them to Randolph.

Randy called daily, hour-long calls. He threatened to fly over to conduct business in person, to help her pack. She vetoed each offer. One minute he vowed that he loved her, begging her to come home. The next he gloated on his position, making certain that Sydney knew he was handling the job well.

In between, he questioned what was delaying her return. "Is there someone else?" he had asked. "Are you chasing your rainbows? . . . What would your father say about neglecting your responsibilities at Barrington Enterprises?" With a breath barely taken, he had asked, "Are you planning to move Barrington's headquarters to the English countryside?"

Sydney swung Abigail's desk chair around and looked out on the Windrush. She was at home here—as comfortable in her leather pumps as she was in her bare feet by the river. A country girl, a city girl, all in one, her father had called her.

But more and more Randolph sounded like the professional side of her father: arrogant, assertive, superior. Through her new image of Randy, her father was toppling from his pedestal. She dangled the receiver between her thumb and forefinger and dropped it in its cradle, severing the connection completely.

Still she heard her own words echoing in the empty room. "All right, Randy. I'll see to a reservation this week. I'll be home soon. Just go ahead with the government contract for more jet fighters. You're authorized to sign in my absence."

"I already did," he had announced as the call ended.

Randy knew how to hit and hit hard. She had not shirked her job by conducting the business of Barrington Enterprises from her makeshift office in the Broadshire library. Never had she been happier than in this temporary control center in the heart of the Cotswolds. But were her decisions linked to the presence of Commander Willoughby in Stow-on-the-Woodland?

Yes, dear Randolph, in my wild fantasies, I have considered moving the main office to England.

She sat for another ten minutes before wandering outside where she found Abigail and Keeley sitting by the fountain. In that moment, she saw herself as a six-year-old, crying because she was going back to America. The sound of the water stirred another memory. Jonas had not wanted her to go away back then.

Keeley fled to her side. She sat down and felt the comfort of the child against her, much as she had felt comforted on Abigail's lap so many years ago. "Abigail, just this moment, I truly remembered being here as a child. I'll have so many memories to take home with me."

"Must you go?"

"Soon. Randolph insists."

"Is Mr. Iverson that important to you?"

"We were engaged once."

"And did you love him?"

"I don't think so. Not really. He was good to me when my parents died. He was their choice. But, he is so like Aaron. Strong willed. Dominant."

"Jonas is strong willed."

"Not in the same way. Jonas, tough as he is, is tethered with kindness. He set aside his career for you and the Admiral."

"He'll go back on sea duty soon. And we'll all miss him, especially you, Sydney. But, dear child, you come from separate worlds. Different backgrounds. Different beliefs."

"So did Millicent and Aaron, but they loved each other."

"Yes, I disapproved of Aaron, but he did love her."

"And, Abigail, your children all came from different backgrounds and beliefs. And you loved them."

"Yes," she said. "From my very first boys. Hermann and Isaac are grown men now. Fathers and grandfathers themselves. They're living in Israel. I hear from them at Hanukkah and on my birthday. Now and then, Hermann surprises me with a phone call."

"They were a big responsibility."

"But never a burden. They were like my own. I always had the hope of Neil coming home and the four of us being a family. Just knowing they are well now pleases me." She laughed, a deep, bubbling chuckle. "By the end of the war, I had five more children in my care—five evacuees from the London blitz."

"You were only a child yourself."

"Yes, not quite twenty-three when the war ended. Neil was gone by then, so Edmund Gallagher's father helped me through the legal battle of sending Hermann and Isaac to a kibbutz in Israel. Emigrating to Israel was what the boys wanted, but I hated sending them away. Within weeks, three of the other children went home to London, and Social Services sent the other two to orphanages in Cornwall. For a time I had no children at all."

Keeley had listened in silence. Abigail patted her knee. "Keeley, little children have always come to live with me."

Sydney hugged the child on her lap. "Abigail, I can't imagine how you supported all of them in wartime."

"Lady Willoughby's parents came to my rescue. Helen was still a child herself—Helen Broadshire back then. Her parents made certain that my children didn't go hungry. I never asked how they managed ration cards for us. Helping us seemed to be their bit for the war. I was given the task of a parlor maid; it meant beds and food for the boys and girls even though we had to live in the servants' quarters beneath the south wing. The boys liked being close to the gun gallery. Helen liked coming down for visits. We became great friends—at least we were friends then."

A gray cloud swept across her face, an undefined sadness. "I left their employ after the children were gone and went back to school. But I was old for my years." She laughed, the same soft ripple. "I think war and motherhood does that to you."

She rested and went on. "When I finally went back to the manor, the older Broadshires had died and left the place to Lady Helen. I had seen little of her in those intervening years. She went to boarding school and finishing school and did a season or two in London. That's where she met the Admiral. He was several years older, but once Helen set her eyes on him, that was it."

A faraway smile touched her face. "It was Sir James who opened the door when I went back to the manor looking for a job. A tall, handsome naval officer. A commanding man even then. He never lifted an eyebrow when I told him I had children with me."

"And you stayed on ever since?"

"Yes. Griselda was part of the kitchen staff then—the same gruff yet warm and caring woman that you know. The children have been a bond between us. She saw me through great difficulties. I shall always be grateful to her for that."

Abigail gazed off toward the hills. Still curious, Sydney asked, "Is it true that you own Broadshire Manor now?"

Abigail's clasped knuckles turned white. "Yes, the manor and all the property surrounding it are legally mine."

"But Jonas has no idea my name is on your will. Edmund Gallagher called me at my summer retreat and told me I had inherited this property. It was all a lie. Why, Abigail?"

Tears balanced on her thick lashes. "I can't tell you what happened. Someday perhaps I will. Edmund is so unlike his father. He has used my deception to his advantage. He doesn't know exactly how I obtained this property, but he is digging for answers. The truth is, I was fighting for my rights. Poor Lady Willoughby! None of us thought she would die so young. But you are right to be concerned. I must rewrite my will before this fluttering heart of mine gives out altogether."

"And will you remove my name?"

"Yes. I know how much you've grown to love this old place, but it belongs to Jonas. I fear not living long enough to rewrite my will. I don't have the strength to face Edmund alone, nor the courage to tell Jonas how I deceived his mother so long ago."

"Changing your will won't please Edmund. He wants to parcel out the land to developers and turn the manor into a showcase."

Her knuckled hands trembled. "That's why I refused to sign the papers on my last appointment—just before my heart attack."

"I have a lawyer friend," said Sydney. "He doesn't know British law, but he won't let Edmund coerce you into signing anything. Jeff might suggest that you settle your affairs right here at the manor. He could make the arrangements."

"A deathbed repentance?" Abigail asked. "Your lawyer friend might put Edmund on the defensive."

"They're already at odds."

Sydney scooted Keeley off her lap. "Go tell Griselda I'm coming for tea. Then Abigail can go to her room and get some rest before supper."

As Keeley left them Abigail said, "I invited Jonas to have supper with me in my room. I plan to tell him what happened the night I had my heart attack. You won't mind eating without us, will you? He thinks I'm hiding Conon here on the property. I don't even know where Conon is." She closed her eyes, her color as gray as it had been moments ago. "Regardless of how Jonas feels, Conon is one of my boys. I'll never forgive myself for sending him away."

"Come, Abby, I'll walk you to your room."

Moments later, relieved to be in her own bed once again, Abigail reached under her pillow and retrieved a medicine bottle. "Tell Griselda that I want her to call Edmund in a few days when I'm feeling stronger. Oh, Sydney, Edmund has caused you great trouble, hasn't he? But I'm glad it brought you to us."

Her eyelids fluttered. "I'd like to take communion before I meet Edmund. Do you think Charles would come and pray with me?"

"I'll ask him while you're sleeping."

Her uneven breathing eased. "When all of these things are settled, I want to spend time with the Admiral again. It takes such a long time to get one's house in order."

At midnight Sydney sat propped on her bed, too pent up for sleep as she listened to the muffled voices of Jonas and Abigail in the next room. A few minutes later a knock came on her door. She pulled her robe around her. "Come in."

Jonas poked his head in. "I saw the light under your door. I'm leaving tomorrow, and I wanted you to know."

"Are we at war again? Abigail said it would take a war to send you back to sea."

He smiled wanly. "I'm flying to Ireland tomorrow afternoon. I'm going back to the place where Louise was killed." His words meshed together. "I have to bring closure to that part of my life—because I care about someone else."

Someone else? Sydney could hear the faint lopping sound of the Windrush. "Jonas, this is not something you should do alone."

"That's how Louise took the trip."

"That was different. She didn't know what would happen. And I don't know what will happen to you if you go alone."

"I can take care of myself. The negotiations in Northern Ireland are coming to a close. We don't expect any more trouble."

"Then why are you so anxious to find Conon O'Reilly?"

"Conon is still trying to prove his own worth by holding to the principles of the IRA. Regardless of the bloodshed."

"Do you go to Ireland with the Navy's blessing?"

"No, but I go with Abigail's. Abigail told me you would want to go with me. Will you go, Sydney?" he asked.

As the jet lowered for a landing, Sydney gazed down on a blue-green lake and the verdant Celtic hills. At the departure gate, Jonas held out his hand to her and led the way through the terminal to the car rental. Driving toward the place where Louise had made the wrong turn, Sydney studied the firm set of his jaw and wondered how long this ruggedly handsome man with his sea- and sun-tanned face could go on wearing a facade of strength. She was there for him. Perhaps in the end that would be enough.

They rode through a countryside carpeted in emerald green, past wet meadows, monastic ruins, and around mist-veiled farmland. In the shadow of the glen where cattle and sheep grazed, they came to a whitewashed farmhouse. Jonas maneuvered the car over a rough road toward a woodsy area with charred undergrowth.

As he stepped from the car, he unfolded a crudely sketched map. "This is it, Sydney. I'm going on alone."

She watched him trudge several feet before stopping beneath an old shade tree with drooping limbs. He stood—a tall, proud man, facing his grief. He was wearing dark slacks and a Shetland sweater, but she pictured him in his uniform, his officer's cap in the crook of his arm, offering a final salute to the woman he had wanted to marry.

Tufts of his raven hair caught in the gentle breeze, and the emerald hills engulfed him. In a way this was a memorial service to his dead fiancée as he worked out his good-bye and fought his unending battle against unknown assailants. At sea—in the midst of a major crisis and as squadron leader—he had not flown home for her funeral. She wondered now whether he ever cried for Louise. Or would the Admiral frown at tears coming from his son?

She saw his shoulder jerk. Once, twice. She went to him and slipped her arm in his. The leaves in the tree rustled. A bird's clear sweet notes mocked their silence.

Sydney heard the rickety, donkey-drawn cart before she saw it barreling over the field toward them. The driver with a weather-scarred face pulled to a stop near them. The cart wheels blew an unexpected cloud of dust from the ground, the breeze wafting the smell of a wagon load of peat toward them.

"A good day to you. I'm Sean Callahan." He squinted down at them from beneath his battered straw hat, a man perhaps in his late sixties. "You're on my property, so I ask you to be leaving."

Sydney tugged at Jonas's arm. "Let's get out of here."

He studied their faces. "No need if you be needing help."

"I'm Jonas Willoughby. My fiancée was killed here three years ago, Mr. Callahan."

"In that car bombing?" Unexpected sympathy shadowed the faded gray eyes. "You're the first ones to come asking after her. A clergyman's daughter according to the news accounts."

As Callahan climbed down from his cart, Sydney pulled at Jonas's arm again. "Let's go, Jonas."

The Irishman removed his hat and beckoned them to follow. He led them through a grove of trees to a cleared space of land. A bouquet of wilted flowers lay propped against a charred tree.

"It happened yonder. Blew the trees out. Blew the car apart. Killed the lass instantly. . . . Not likely she knew." He rubbed his forearm across his eyes. "My daughter died the same way in that bombing in Omagh, so we know how you be feeling."

"No one knows how I feel," Jonas said, but he was in control. "Were you here when it happened, sir?"

"I was at my wife's bedside at the hospital. I refused to trust her life in the hands of Protestant doctors in Belfast."

Jonas nodded toward the farm. "Then the house was empty?"

The battered hat shaded his solemn eyes again. "No, I left my son-in-law and his friends in charge of the farm. Never should have done that. Thought I could trust them for that long."

Jonas winced. "Was your son-in-law involved in the bombing?"

"No proof," Callahan said. "But I know how his mind works. We never wanted Rorie to marry him. But our Rorie was going to have his child, and my wife couldn't stand the shame."

Keeley, Sydney thought. *He's talking about Keeley O'Reilly.*

He gave a feeble sweep of his hand. "It was days before they cleared the mess away. The grass has grown back, but I'll be dead before we can replace the trees and see them grow tall like they were. Mrs. Callahan puts those flowers there—for your fiancée and for our daughter. So senseless, these killings."

Say something, Jonas, Sydney thought. *Mr. Callahan is reaching out to you. He's hurting too.* She pressed his arm.

"Thank your wife for me. Sir, is your son-in-law here now?"

The wrinkled face hardened. "I ordered him off the property after the accident. Told him to be gone, to never come back." His mouth twisted. "His friends were responsible for your fiancée's death. They fled before the police arrived. The police found my son-in-law up at the farm, napping with his two children."

Jonas glowered. "He slept through the explosion?"

Another twisted grimace cut through the Irishman's wrinkles. "Would you have slept through it, Mr. Willoughby?"

"No. Never."

"Don't know why I ever took them in. Guess I thought my son-in-law would reform for the sake of his children."

"I'd like to get in touch with him."

"He's not worth the search. He laughed in my face the day he left. Told me they'd be hiding out in various places until the last peace agreement is signed—and then they will strike again."

He rubbed his eyes once more. "The peace we prayed for could be destroyed. We won't even know who they are or where they are. I'd like the hatred to end in my lifetime."

"Sir, it's apt to get worse before it gets better."

"I know," he said wearily. "There's a song in my country that only our rivers run free. But I'd like things settled in my lifetime so my daughter's death will have some purpose. So my poor wife can have some peace."

"The conflict will come to an end someday, sir."

"I wish I shared your confidence, young man. Better if I had turned in my daughter's husband when I had the chance. If I had to do it over, I would have shot him myself."

"Revenge never works, sir. I should know."

The wrinkles in the old man's face seemed permanently embedded by pain and weather. "He's out there somewhere, still looking for a home for his children. He wanted my wife to raise them. I wouldn't hear of it. Didn't need any reminders of my Rorie."

He walked back to the donkey cart and pointed toward the end of the road. "I told my daughter's husband to get out and to take his children with him. They looked like him. The youngest only an infant then. If only they had looked more like Rorie." He shrugged helplessly. "My wife has never forgiven me for sending our grandchildren away."

Someday, Sydney thought, *I'll bring them back and let you hold them again. You'll see how much like Rorie they really are.*

240

She patted his hand. "There's still time for your grand-children to grow up without bloodshed. Maybe your son-in-law will realize that. Maybe he will change."

"No. Not that lad. I told Rorie he was no good when she ran off with him. But I have to give the devil his due. He loves those children of his." Callahan went back to pick up the wilted flowers. "I'll have my wife replace these. It's all we can do. We still feel responsible for that poor lass turning off on the wrong road—getting herself killed like that."

Jonas looked gaunt. "Louise always had trouble reading maps and often made the wrong turns on the motorway."

"Pity. You can't see them now, but there were tire tracks where she tried to turn the car around. My son-in-law's friends were too quick for her. I knew when that happened that they had used my place for an arsenal—a place for building bombs."

Sydney shuddered. "The police never arrested anyone?"

"Been three years. They wouldn't be looking now. Even the local police aren't wanting to stir up trouble. We're a peaceful people here. All my wife and I ever wanted to do was raise crops and make a home for our grandchildren."

"But you sent them away."

His voice turned gravelly, belligerent. "Had to. Keeping them spelled trouble. We're a Catholic neighborhood. A few kilometers over, the Protestants settled in. We want no disfavor with them."

"How old are your grandchildren?" Sydney asked. She felt Jonas's eyes turn on her, but she kept her face averted.

"Danny would be about three. The girl two years older."

Jonas stiffened. The farmer nodded toward his cart filled with peat. "I need to be getting this fuel back to the house. Would you be liking to come in for some Irish beer?"

"No thank you. No beer of any kind," Jonas told him.

"Then some Irish coffee?" he said with a twinkle.

"We'll pass on that one too. We have a plane to catch."

"The papers said the girl was engaged to a Harrier pilot."

241

The muscles in Jonas's jaw grew taut. He stretched out his hand to the farmer. "The newspapers don't always get their facts straight. Thank you for taking time to talk to us. I could never bring myself to come before this—"

"Too busy flying those jets?"

"Busy," Jonas acknowledged. "It was good to see that the ground cover is growing in again. I don't think I could have faced it if the ground were still charred."

The man took his battered hat off again. "With your fiancée's father being a vicar, would he want us to pray here? You likely belong to them Protestants, but maybe you'd like to say a little prayer here for your fiancée."

When Jonas hesitated, Sydney said, "That would be nice."

The farmer's craggy face lit with understanding. "Maybe you're a bit rusty along those lines. No matter. I think we all have a hook in the Lord's Prayer." He twirled his old cap and closed his heavy lids. "Our Father," he began in a tremulous voice.

Jonas joined him. "Hallowed be thy name . . . forgive us . . ."

Unsure of the words, Sydney kept her own prayer to a soft murmur. "Deliver us from evil—" *Deliver me from evil.*

She heard the farmer's footsteps as he left, heard the labored breathing as he climbed back on the donkey cart loaded with smelly peat. When they opened their eyes, he lifted his battered cap to them and was gone.

Jonas took her hand. "I thought I was bearing the weight of the world until I met that man. He's a giant, isn't he?"

"But he turned his grandchildren away."

"He did what he thought was best for his community."

"When he turned that cart toward the farmhouse, he was telling us it was time to leave. He wanted us to go away and not come back. But, Jonas, I should like to come again and meet his wife. We must bring Danny and Keeley back someday."

"So you know who he is? You can come back, Sydney, but don't ask me to come with you. You see, I knew who Callahan was before we came. Captain McIntyre traced Conon's family ties here. I came here to say good-bye to Louise, but I also came on that slim chance of finding Conon O'Reilly hiding out here."

At the car, he took another glance back at the place where Louise had lost her life. The emerald island never seemed more peaceful. "If Louise had chosen a place to die, it would have been here. She loved Ireland and wanted to share it with me."

"She just did."

Sydney glanced up, half expecting the sky to reflect the green of the Irish hills. But it was a powdery blue, with broken patches of wispy clouds drifting lazily above them.

"Sydney, it would have pleased Louise that you came here with me. She never wanted me to be alone."

Twenty-three

Gregor sat on the ground, hugging his bare knees to his chest. As Jonas placed flowers in a tin of water, Gregor asked, "Are they for Louise?"

Jonas nodded. He glanced down at the freshly cut flowers. Primroses with their buds still tight, the brilliant clump of green-winged orchids, the last of the sweet-scented jasmine that Louise had always loved. It struck him that he should be cutting flowers for Sydney Barrington. Courting the living, not still mourning the dead. He faced the boy again.

Gregor's shoes pointed inward, toeing the grass—a sure sign that he was upset, warding off rejection.

"May I go down to the cemetery with you, Jonas?"

"Not this time. I want to talk to Reverend Charles on a personal matter."

"About Miss Sydney?"

The boy's perception annoyed him. Jonas snapped off one more orchid. "She might come into the conversation." More kindly, he added, "Charles and I often speak about you."

Gregor's eyes brightened, lustrous dark circles in a childish face. "Why?"

"He wants you to sing in the choir when school begins."

"With Tesa and Keeley? I'd rather go to boarding school."

"I told him we're planning a trip to Gordonstoun so you can visit my school. I went there when I was eight."

He watched Gregor's boldness vanish. Was Gregor at nine too young, too vulnerable to send away to boarding school?

"We'll wait until you see the place before we decide. And then we'll have to convince Miss Sydney that you are man enough to go away."

"Sydney was looking for you."

"She was?" He automatically gave his corduroys and shirt a once-over. Brushing the soil from his hands, he glanced toward the front door. "When?"

"When her and Keeley went horseback riding."

"She and Keeley," he corrected. "I don't think you like Miss Barrington much, do you?"

"Mrs. Quigley says she wants to sell Broadshire Manor."

"It's not for sale, Gregor."

"But if she does, you will go away?"

"You know I'm going back to sea someday. We've talked about it." He ruffled the boy's hair and grabbed up the tin of flowers. "I'll be back in an hour. This afternoon we can gather the sheep in. Maybe walk out on the knoll. You'd like that, wouldn't you?"

"Just the two of us, Jonas?"

He had thought to ask Sydney, but he said, "Of course. Just the two of us. Come on. Walk me to the gate and that's as far as you go. Tell Mrs. Quigley I'll be back for the noon meal."

"Will you take a tray to the Admiral when you come back?"

"If you go with me. He eats better for you, young man."

He left Gregor at the gate and strolled off without looking back. Why had the boy latched on to him, making going back to sea more difficult? Even this morning, Griselda had told him, "I don't take kindly to what you're doing to that boy. Having him eat out of your hand. Following you everywhere. I don't understand the likes of you, Jonas Willoughby. Coming home like you did. Taking over. Gregor will fall apart when you go away."

Life seemed muddied enough. Why did it have to include an orphan boy from Kosovo? *How could I even think to court*

Sydney Barrington with the boy on one heel and TopGun on the other?

He knew that Griselda's snarl was a cover-up. It was her feeble defense at the thought of him turning over the manor to the National Trust and going back to sea. Didn't she understand? He would make provisions for her and the children. But she wanted life to go on as it always had. The running of the house was her realm. She rarely welcomed anyone in her kitchen even to boil a kettle of water for tea. Not even when the tea was for Abigail.

Life on board the carrier had been far simpler.

When Jonas reached the Church of St. Michael's, he found Charles walking in the churchyard and humming one of Louise's favorite hymns about angels guarding and defending us. He marveled at the man with all of his losses still singing. Jonas had long ago laid aside his own melody.

"Good morning, Charles."

He turned, not seeing for a moment, and then the song on his lips died. "Jonas, you came early today."

"I brought flowers." He felt as though the flowers for Louise were merely an offering to pave the way for other things. They took the few steps to the grave site together. Jonas stooped down and arranged the flowers in the tin of water.

Charles knelt on one knee. "She would have liked those, but I think you are here with something else on your mind."

For a second time within a half hour, Jonas found himself brushing soil from his hands. "I wanted to talk to you about Sydney Barrington. You see, lately, I just can't get her out of my mind."

If the announcement shocked Charles, he hid his reaction. "Sounds like matters of the heart from the look on your face."

They stood, the older man almost losing his balance. "Should we walk out here, Jonas, or do you wish to go inside the church?"

"Not in the sanctuary. This is not a spiritual matter," he blurted. "Not a confession." And yet as he said the words, it was both. "I only need a moment of your time."

He had talked to Charles about growing older, had thought of him as living in the twilight years. Suddenly the man aged before his eyes. His face seemed a maze of wrinkles, the tired eyes without merriment. His mouth sagged, aging him even more. But Charles reached out and put his broad hands on Jonas's shoulders. They felt strong and manly, the grip ageless.

His voice remained steady. "Are you in love with her?"

"I don't know, Charles." He stared down at the tombstone.

Louise Rainford-Simms
Beloved daughter
Lost in Ireland; alive in Jesus

His gaze veered off toward the hills and slowly back to Charles. "I thought there would never be anyone after Louise."

"Surely Louise would understand," Charles said, his voice quivering. He turned abruptly and strode into the house.

Jonas caught up with him in the sitting room and found Charles bending over his electric trains. The train set had been built from scratch and run by a generator so the diocese would not complain of needless costs at the vicarage. The hobby had always been a source of pleasure to Charles, a great comfort to him at Louise's death. Now in Stow-on-the-Woodland, it was the chance for the children of the village to come to the vicarage to hear about the Shepherd.

Charles examined the caboose on the freight train and placed it back on the track. As he did so, a tear splashed on the rails. "We could talk about this another time," Jonas said quietly.

"No, it's long past time to bare our thoughts to each other. You've avoided me since you came home. Perhaps I have been avoiding this meeting."

247

He repositioned the railroad crossings and the depot and gave a little twist to the toy church with a steeple. "I call it St. James after my last parish." He looked up at last. "I've been watching you and Miss Barrington strolling over the knolls and walking together by the river. When I shut my eyes, I imagine that it is Louise and you again. Pretending what happened didn't happen. It's just—seeing you come with the flowers and knowing now that you won't be doing that any longer."

His eyes misted with more unshed tears. "Forgive me, Jonas. These are just the rambling thoughts of an old man. I long ago came to terms about my daughter's death. I realize now that I had not come to terms with having the man she loved fall in love again."

He held up his hand. "No, Jonas. Let me go on. I thought for years that this might happen. But I thought you would be away somewhere. At Portsmouth or in Paris. And you'd post me a letter saying you had married. I could have wept in private then."

"You're Abigail's minister. I thought I should come to you."

"You were part of St. Michael's parish when you were a boy and even when you were courting Louise. It's good that you came to me. Sit down. I'll have Kersten bring us some tea."

Jonas sat and crossed his lanky legs.

The reverend's skin turned red above the clerical collar. "After we lost Louise, you changed, Jonas. I saw it in your eyes. In the set curve of your mouth. I couldn't see your heart, but I knew it was hardened. Mine was like that for weeks after her death." He smiled, his watery eyes brimming. "You have been like a son to me since the day my daughter brought you here. Do you remember what she said that first Sunday afternoon?"

"I remember. I was shocked, in fact."

He mimicked his daughter. "'Father, this Navy boy may be an old reprobate, but I love him. I'm going to marry him when he gets around to asking me.' What a wicked little charmer she was. You were a happy pair. And then—Ireland came between us. I want you to be happy again, but you must understand. Louise was my daughter. The one who brought me my greatest happiness after my wife's death."

Jonas allowed his gaze to sweep the familiar room. A smoke-blackened kettle dangled over the stone fireplace. The painting of the Garden of Gethsemane hung above the mantel, its frame warped on one corner. The ancient chairs felt uncomfortable, as though sitting stiffly in them brought humility to the shepherd of St. Michael's. He allowed himself the pain of stealing a glimpse of the portrait of Louise that sat on the console table.

Jonas's attention was drawn back to Charles as Kersten poured tea for them. She smiled sweetly at Jonas, a young woman around Louise's age with rose-colored lips that looked good on her and brows finely plucked above those curious dark eyes.

"It's safe to try the biscuits, Commander Willoughby. Mrs. Quigley made them." She sashayed from the room, her long hair bouncing on her narrow shoulders.

"I see what Mrs. Quigley meant now. Kersten doesn't look the part of a housekeeper, Charles."

"There's plenty of space in the old vicarage for lonely people to wander around. She hasn't made many friends since coming to the village, and it's hard for me to keep a smiling face seven days a week when people only come by on Sundays."

"And hash out your sermons the rest of the week?"

"Is that what you do, Jonas?"

"Sydney asks a lot of questions. Last week you talked about the sympathizing Jesus—and Sydney kept asking me who He was."

Charles tented his fingers, a faint smile finding its way to his lips. "That's from a hymn."

"I know, but Sydney didn't. This past Sunday, you worried her about the spotless Lamb. She said she doesn't know Him. You should talk to her."

His fingers remained tented. "Jonas, *you* must tell her about the Lamb. I practice my sermons on Kersten—that way she hears them. She finds herself too busy on Sundays to worship with us."

Most of the village finds something else to do, Jonas thought. But he asked, "Is she busy cooking?"

"Mercy no. She's a much better artist than cook. Of late, though, she's been learning some recipes in Mrs. Quigley's kitchen." He patted his stomach. "So things are tasting better now."

A resounding thump startled them both. "What was that?"

"Perhaps Kersten dropped the kettle again."

But Jonas knew the thumping sounds did not belong to Kersten. "Do you have a guest, Charles?"

"The two friends of Miss Barrington. You've met them at the pub. It means more work for Kersten, but she has taken an interest in the young man from Chicago." Charles leaned his head back, hands clasped. "Kersten came from America. She sees herself as an artist. She's good too. Ought to be," he chuckled. "She paints the same scene over and over. Mostly the golden hills with the Windrush winding through."

"So she won't stay forever?"

"Few of us do, Jonas. She has free room and board for as long as she needs it. She does light housekeeping for me. And now and again, I phone her family to reassure them that she is well."

He switched gears abruptly. "Jonas, have you told Miss Barrington how you feel? One usually goes to the woman he loves, not to the parish priest."

"How can I? We come from two separate worlds." He wiped the palms of his hands on his corduroys. "I can't give up my world."

"Do you expect her to give up hers?"

"That wouldn't be fair either. I remember how lonely my mother was with Dad always away at sea."

"I would not worry too much about Miss Barrington giving up her own career. She is determined to carry on her father's defense company until she can turn it over to a reliable staff. But I think she came here as much to find herself as to lay claim to Broadshire Manor. She's found her way into the hearts of several of us."

Mine mostly, Jonas thought.

"Has she considered basing her company here in Europe? Other corporations have done so. If she wins the contract for the carriers, she'd have more of a reason to remain in England."

"I can't ask her to do that."

"You won't have to. She's untangling the threads of her life. Give her time, Jonas. Louise would be happy for you."

The silence dragged as Charles refilled their cups. "I came here about something else, Charles. Something I haven't had the courage to face before. You see—I feel responsible for what happened to Louise."

"How could you? You weren't even there."

"Charles, why in the name of heaven—"

"Be careful, son."

"What possessed her to go on our honeymoon trip alone?"

Charles looked up, his bushy white brows arching. "Son, she loved you, but it humiliated her to cancel the wedding plans. She had to get away."

"My ship was going right out—a quick turnaround with deployment back to the Adriatic. There was no time to bring in another pilot. I thought Louise understood."

"I think she realized that day that your career would always come first with you. That you would never give up the Service. She was like her mother, God rest her soul. Louise needed someone to be with her. All she really wanted was a home, a hearth, a fireplace. She wanted to curl up beside you."

His cup rattled as he put it on the saucer. "As you know, about the time of your engagement, the diocese offered me a choice between retirement or taking a much neglected parish in Stow-on-the-Woodland. And so I came here. I wanted to be here for Louise during those lonely months when you were at sea."

"Forgive me for failing your daughter."

"You didn't fail her. I did. I fed into her fancies. I thought that once you were married—once you had a child—you might resign your commission and come home to stay."

"I never told her that."

"I know. But she believed in her own charms. She was convinced the Admiral had influenced your choice of the Navy."

"I wanted the Navy for myself. I had to fly. I remember the first time I watched a ship sail from Portsmouth. The first time I flew solo. It's in my blood."

"When you had to cancel the wedding, she knew that the Navy would always come first with you. That's why she went ahead with the trip to Ireland. She wanted to work things out for herself."

"The day I heard—" Jonas tried again. "The day I heard she had been killed, my world fell apart. She meant everything to me, Charles."

"If she had given me the choice, I would have chosen you for a son-in-law. You're trustworthy. Hard-working. And what pleased me most was that you genuinely loved my daughter."

Jonas choked out the words. "I never meant her to go to Ireland without me. I should have been with her."

"And then I would have lost both of you in that bombing."

Heavy footsteps resounded on the other side of the parish wall. Jonas frowned. "I'm telling you; it sounds like that noise is coming through the paneling."

The reverend's expression turned anxious. "That's the way it is in this old vicarage. Dank and cold and full of ghosts."

Jonas was certain he was not teasing. "I should go and let you get some rest."

"Yes, do that."

He stood and watched Charles rise wearily in front of him. Again the cleric planted his broad hands on Jonas's shoulders. But this time his hands trembled. "We shall talk again, Jonas. And you have my blessing, whatever decision you make."

Charles stared into empty space for several minutes, then he slid back the panel and stepped into the Jacobean chamber with his prayer book in his hands. The stench of decaying flesh filled his nostrils. Old dressings stained with blood and pus lay on the floor. He had come into the room to confront the young man lying helplessly on the cot and felt only pity as Lucas sponged the feverish body.

"Lucas, the boy needs a doctor."

"And ruin my position with the Admiral? No. It won't be long. One way or the other, I will have him out of here."

Conon's words seemed strangled as he said, "We heard you talking, Charles. I didn't know about your daughter. I didn't know she was Jonas's fiancée."

"Her death almost destroyed him. After my daughter died, his career was all that mattered to him."

Conon's shallow breathing turned raspy. "That sounds like Jonas. Unblemished commitment and loyalty to the British crown. And those bloody bagpipes? Is he still playing them?"

"Sometimes, out on the hills. Conon, it's been three years since Louise was killed—on a farm not far from Belfast."

"My wife died the same way." Conon struggled to go on speaking. "I didn't know your daughter died in an IRA ambush. I'm sorry. You've been so kind to me—" He thrashed on the bed, fought for coherence again. "I heard the bomb go off, sir."

Stunned, Charles gripped the boy's shoulder and shook him. "What are you saying?"

"Careful, Reverend," Lucas warned.

"Conon, what are you saying?" Sudden rage consumed Charles. He gripped Conon's arm. "Were you there when my daughter died?"

The red-flushed eyes opened again as Lucas left the room. "My wife's father owned the farm. I went there to ask him to make a home for my children. But when that girl was killed, even their grandfather turned my children away."

His grip tightened. "Did you kill my daughter?"

Conon blinked his bloodshot eyes. "My friends did."

Charles fought his rage. "Why, Conon O'Reilly? She never did a thing to you. What a fool I have been offering you refuge."

"It's your job, isn't it? To help the sick and dying."

The prayer book almost slipped from his hand. "Get out. You're nothing but trouble, Mr. O'Reilly."

Conon tried to pull himself to a sitting position. "Lucas promises to get me out of here soon. We told you all along that once I could walk, I'd be gone. Now Lucas plans to fly me out."

"Fly you out? He has no access to a plane."

"He promises to find one."

"Lucas has no intention of risking his own safety for you, Conon. Let me go for Dr. Wallis. Let me turn you in for the sake of your children." His anger was a mixture of mercy and pain. "Don't ruin the peace negotiations by taking up arms again."

"I'm sorry about your daughter. You have to believe me. Just give me a few days, Reverend. I want to see my children one more time before I leave."

"If I arrange it, will you go away?"

254

"Yes. I'll leave on my own if I have to—if I can just see my children one more time."

"Miss Barrington takes the children for walks every day, usually before the noon meal. You can see them then."

He swayed on the narrow cot. "If I'm caught doing so, it could ruin you, Reverend."

"Yes, I would have to resign."

For hours after he left the Jacobean room, Charles roamed the hills and searched his own soul. It would be so easy to call Jonas back—to take him to the narrow room and tell him, "There. There's the man who watched your fiancée die."

Out on the wolds, he talked to the sympathizing Jesus, begging for understanding and mercy and knowing that he must show mercy to the dying man. At midnight he came to terms with his own pain. He would not—could not—turn a man from the church.

St. Michael's is your house, dear God, he reasoned, *and the young terrorist is a prodigal who fears dying and longs for peace.*

Twenty-four

As Sydney tossed on her canopy bed, the urgency that had sent her flying to England invaded her subconscious, forcing her into sleeplessness. Abigail Broderick needed her. The undefined cry for help exploded in Sydney's ears. It echoed louder than the rumble of the Windrush. Blew in stronger than the breeze rustling the curtains of her open window. Cried out full-throated like the screech of the night owl.

Thumping her pillows and shifting her tired body, she tacked the demands of her life on an imaginary clipboard. Her staff at Barrington Enterprises was capable of carrying out her orders. But if she wiggled her toes in Aaron Barrington's shoes, he would expect her to take the brunt of leadership—not allow someone else to do it. These demands weighed against the needs in the Cotswolds; the unsolved problems at Broadshire Manor: the handsome pilot who wanted nothing more than to go back to sea; the five-year-old who had wrapped her very existence around Sydney's heartstrings; Abigail's failing health and her unswerving loyalty to the Admiral and to the Irishman who had come to her for help and left his children behind.

The choice was Sydney's. She could stay on in this quiet hamlet of Stow-on-the-Woodland or return to the chaotic rush of life back home. She flung back the bedcovers and pulled on her warm khaki slacks and university sweatshirt to ward off the chill of the pre-dawn hours. Opening her suitcase, she found her mother's dolls tucked in with her heavy socks and running shoes. The rag doll in denim overalls and the empress doll dressed in taffeta and lace. The doll she was to give to someone special.

She put the dolls against the pillows on the side where Keeley would crawl in and wait for her return. Then she crept past Abigail's room, felt her way safely to the massive front door, and let herself out. The gate creaked as she slipped through, jangled as it swung closed again. She felt no fear in the pre-dawn mist, no apprehension at being alone. The light drizzle of rain that had tapped against her windows during the night had left the fresh after-scent of a spring rain on the meadows. Within minutes she was on the footpath, making her way through the woodland down to the Windrush.

As dawn began to break, she dropped to the bank, hugged her knees to her chest, and sat there thrilling to the river tumbling beneath the bridge. The verges along the riverbank swayed back and forth. The cottonwoods and weeping willows dripped the dew of morning. The cottages became more than shadows until inch by inch the glow of dawn turned the hills golden and night disappeared completely. With it came the awakening of the birds and the sweet scent of flowers opening their buds to the morning.

Now she saw St. Michael's through the trees and two men walking there together. She recognized Charles at once but not the other man. He was leaning heavily against the vicar and was almost carried by him into the parish.

Charles saw Sydney and took a steadying grip on Conon's arm. "Come, Conon. We must get you back inside."

"Why?" His speech slurred. "I need air. I'm having more difficulty breathing. I don't want to go back in there."

"The minute you stepped into the vicarage, you became my responsibility."

"Would your archbishop see it that way, Reverend?"

He chuckled. "We do have a difference of opinion from time to time."

"Is that what landed you here in this little village?"

"My age did that. My usefulness to the diocese ran thin."

Conon stopped his halting steps. "You won't get in trouble because of me?"

"I trust not. But each man must live by his conscience."

"I have none, Reverend."

"Perhaps it is just asleep for now."

"I don't understand you forgiving me when your daughter—"

"I'm in the business of forgiveness. You will have to trust me, Conon. That young woman down by the Windrush saw two of us."

"Does it matter?" he asked wearily. "I will never be well enough to leave. Never free enough to see my children again."

"There is one way to see them."

Conon coughed, his chest sounding even more congested this morning. "I couldn't even pick Danny up now. And Keeley saw her mother die in Omagh. She must not see me. I look terrible."

"Conon, you have an infection. You're burning up. Let me send for the doctor or drive you to the hospital. Lucas doesn't have to know."

"Lucas will get me out of here as soon as I can walk."

"You can't even stand alone."

"I will soon." But he went up the steps and through the door leaning hard against the vicar, his body too weak to walk alone.

"Reverend, don't send me behind those walls again. I am sick of that dark room."

"I have no other place to hide you, son. We have guests. The church of the fifteenth century must have planned that room for you."

Charles felt the burning of the young man's body resting against his arm. "Reverend, give me a little longer. I can't stand it behind those walls. This isn't the Chastleton House. Cromwell's men aren't storming the place."

Charles eased his charge down on the couch in his study. "Son, you are a fugitive in this village. I can't guarantee your safety until you go back into the Jacobean room. But rest here for now until Kersten can make you some tea and boil you an egg. She can help you back to your room after you eat."

"No food. I'm not hungry."

"But you must eat."

Conon shivered, his fever rising; Charles pulled a blanket over his legs. "I'm going to leave you here. You must stay quiet. My guests are not to be disturbed."

"Where are you going, Reverend?"

He smiled. "To see another prodigal."

Sydney was still sitting by the Windrush when he reached her and sat down beside her. For several minutes they were silenced by the gentle flow of the river. He stretched his legs toward the water, bracing himself with his palms against the ground.

Finally, he said, "You're up early, Miss Barrington."

"And you?"

"I am accustomed to walking these hills early each morning. I feel closer to God when I do."

"Who was that walking with you?"

He crooked the corner of his mouth. "A young man in need."

"In need of shelter?"

"We all have need of shelter. You have come to the river early this morning. You must have big problems. How may I help you?"

"Is that another one of your morning chores?"

He snuggled into his warm sweater and looked toward the hills. "My parishioners are not always in the pew. This is a peaceful place—an outdoor cathedral. I think that is why you came down here at dawn."

"I'm leaving soon. I came here with so many questions. Now that I'm here, I have a thousand more. I'm worried about the children, particularly the O'Reillys. If something happens to Abigail, Danny and Keeley will be even more lost than they are now. I could take Keeley home with me, but how? Danny would be left behind. They don't even have passports."

"As I said, you have big problems." His attempt to smile was surely mirroring her own unhappiness.

"Do you know what I think, Reverend Rainford-Simms? I think Keeley's father didn't just vanish."

"We discussed that once before, didn't we?" *I have sleepless nights over that,* he thought.

"I still think someone is hiding Conon O'Reilly right here in this village. So it wouldn't be right for me to take Keeley away. It wouldn't be right for me to separate the children."

"Do you not have room in your heart for both of them?"

"Keeley's the first child who ever—oh, if only I knew who was hiding their father, I would persuade him to turn O'Reilly in for the sake of Danny and Keeley."

"Do you have someone in mind?" he asked guardedly.

"Do you want the truth?" She didn't wait for his answer. "I still think you know exactly where he is. This morning—a few moments ago, I had every reason to believe that I was right. Maybe you and Abigail planned this together. Or maybe you helped out because she was so ill. Abigail is gaining some strength—but for how long? But it's the children whose lives are being torn in so many directions."

Charles felt drawn to this sensitive young woman. Felt concern for the turmoil and search that goaded her. From all she had told him during their times together, she seemed to see herself as one living with a handful of memories, a large bank account, and the position of CEO in an ever-expanding global market. All it had done for her was make her feel old at thirty. Here in the Cotswolds she was on the verge of happiness. Yet he found himself wanting her to leave. Not because she was getting close to the truth, but because she obviously was falling in love with Jonas. He fought their friendship, screaming in protest that it was unfair. Jonas belonged to Louise.

What a selfish man you are, Charles, he told himself. *Louise would want Jonas to be happy again.*

He couldn't meet her eyes as he said, "If you are so anxious to go home, you must regret coming here?"

"No. I've been peaceful here, as though the answers for which I've searched all of my life lie just beyond the next hill. But I feel like one of those sheep grazing aimlessly, unable to find my way back without someone to guide me."

He reached up and felt his clerical collar, the symbol of his ministry. He felt as if it was choking him. He should call this hillside a pulpit and tell her of a greater Shepherd. His voice sounded unreal as he said, "I think the answer you want is closer than the next hill. Christ went the distance for you, Sydney Barrington. Why don't you consider Him?"

"I don't want to bother Him with so many things happening. My old fiancé keeps calling and begging me to come home. My engineers are finalizing the blueprints for the carriers so we can bid on that job. And I've scheduled a dinner meeting in London with the British Defense Secretary as my guest. Jonas was shocked when I told him about the dinner."

"What Jonas Willoughby thinks matters to you. I think you see some of the qualities in Jonas that my daughter saw. He's a good man. I'm going to ask you what I asked my daughter a long time ago. Have you told Jonas what's on your heart?"

"And make a fool of myself?"

"Isn't that better than losing him altogether?"

"I think he's worried about everything at the manor, particularly about Abigail. They're quite close, you know."

"Have you ever wondered why?"

"He told me she's always been there for him, especially after his mother died. He really respects her."

"And rightfully so," Charles said.

"They're much alike. Even his smile reminds me of Abigail."

The sun cast its shadow across her cheeks. "So you've noticed the likeness between them?" he asked.

She looked at him sharply. But he knew she saw only innocence in his expression.

"I think she would have liked children of her own, Reverend. Taking in all of those hidden children like she did."

"Yes." Charles tugged at a blade of grass on the riverbank. The sun was higher now, the weather warmer. The Windrush crystal clear. A swan and her ducklings swam across the water. "Mothers tend to protect their young, even when they grow up, Sydney."

"That's the way Abigail has been with all the children. Especially with Jonas. She always jokes and says she has a thousand reasons to love him."

He sat taller and brushed the palms of his big hands. "Have you ever considered the one reason why she really does? The answers are there for you; they are there for Jonas as well. But first Jonas must rid himself of his bitterness against the Irish Republican Army. And you, my dear, must remember that Christ went the distance for you. Once you settle who this Christ is, then everything else will fall into place."

"And then I'll know whether to go home or whether to stay on here in Stow-on-the-Woodland?"

"One answer at a time. I found my greatest happiness here. I always took pride in having a large parish. Did you know? I used to be the Bishop of Monkton in the best of my days, but now I am content to be the Vicar of Stow-on-the-Woodland."

"Oh, I didn't know. I thought you were always here."

"Like the hills?"

She glanced at her watch. "I promised Abigail that we'd spend the day together. She's getting up more each day. Her favorite spot is sitting outside by the fountain."

Without asking permission, Charles breathed a quick prayer for Sydney; then he stood and helped her spring to her feet. "We both have a busy schedule today. Tell Abigail I'll try to come by this evening. I've been missing our good visits."

"I'll tell her." She looked up into his face. "Reverend, if that was Conon O'Reilly walking with you this morning, tell him his children miss him. Tell him I'd like to see him."

The lump in his throat was too big to answer her. He watched her sprint away on those long legs in a graceful motion, her chestnut hair bouncing at her neck. *She knows, and this time she did not accuse me. She is bearing the weight of Broadshire Manor on her shoulders, and she's giving me time to make amends. For the sake of the children? Or Abigail? Or?* And this time the sight of her blurred and the collar at his neck seemed unbearably tight as he watched the young American. Miss Barrington had fallen in love with Jonas, and all he could think about was Louise.

"Oh, God," he prayed. "Forgive me. I have broken faith with You—and with those who need my help."

As Sydney hurried back to the manor, she tried to sort through what Charles had said. The prayer that he had prayed on parting was more glowing than the sunrise. It struck her as she reached the gate that he was trying to tell her something about Abigail and Jonas. Something that would help her decide whether to stay a little bit longer.

They looked alike. They smiled alike. No, Jonas looked like his father with his thick black hair and blue eyes and that stubborn jaw. But he smiled like Abigail.

No, that wasn't it. Abigail had a thousand reasons to love Jonas. No, only one reason, the vicar had said. The thoughts were still troubling Sydney when she found Keeley asleep on her bed, an arm around each doll.

She leaned over and kissed the sleeping child. "Keeley, sweetheart, we're going to have breakfast with Abigail."

Keeley snuggled deeper into the pillow. She could not be roused, so Sydney showered and dressed and went off to find Abigail. At breakfast, at lunch, in the garden, and later as they walked outside and took their places on the bench near the fountain, she searched for words to question Abigail.

One reason. A thousand reasons.

They chatted for long hours. About Jonas. About Lady Willoughby. About Edmund Gallagher and about what Griselda planned to do to him. Abigail spoke, as she always did, gently about the Admiral. In the last few days Sydney had begun to link Abigail Broderick with the frail old man in the west wing. But when Sydney mentioned going home, back to America before another week slipped by, Abigail begged her to say no more.

By late afternoon a southwesterly breeze stirred behind them. Sydney glanced at Abigail. "Would you like to go back in? I don't want you to catch a chill out here."

Abigail shaded her eyes with her rail-thin hand and studied the landscape as the sleepy hamlet waited for the close of another day. "No, let's stay here a while. It's one of my favorite places. I want to watch the sunset."

"Griselda won't like supper getting cold."

"That's one of the good things about my last heart attack. She is letting me set my own pace. We used to keep such a rigid schedule. Besides, I want to be here when Gregor comes home."

"Waiting until all of your children are in! Are you watching for Gregor—or for Jonas?"

She twisted sharply in her chair. "All of my children?"

"That's what you always say, isn't it?" Sydney risked another bold step. "So are you watching for Gregor or for Jonas?"

"I worry about them both." Her words seemed to carry on the wind. "Gregor will be lost when Jonas goes back to sea."

"Did he tell you the *HMS Invincible* is due to dock in Portsmouth next month?"

"I saw the notice in the *Navy News*. And this time I won't try to stop him. He's done so much for us already."

They saw them coming on the high knoll in the distance. Over the rolling hills. Through a patch of wildflowers. Past the winding goat path. Man and boy and TopGun racing ahead of them.

Abigail smiled. *The same smile.* "I must capture that picture of the two of them," she said.

"You must have a hundred such pictures in your mind."

"At least a thousand of Jonas."

So do I, Sydney thought. *And I've only known him for such a little while.* "Jonas is special to you."

"Yes."

Jonas, Abigail. Defined by some invisible cord. Tied together as one. But that could only happen if—if Abigail were his mother. She loved him for a thousand reasons. . . . And I have finally guessed the most important one.

Their voices echoed over the hills. The man's deep chuckle. The boy's shrill laughter. TopGun barking to hurry them along.

"I might not be here when Jonas comes home next time."

Nor I, Sydney thought. "Don't even think that way, Abby."

"If you could feel the uneven flutter in my chest you would understand why I say such things. But your leaving troubles me. Are you running away from Jonas, Sydney?"

"I've left a business unattended far too long."

"Not with all those phone calls and your trips to the Jarrow Shipyard. Didn't I hear you ring long distance this morning?"

She flushed, admitting, "Several times to the States."

"Have you considered keeping your main office in England?"

"Why would I do that?"

"For Jonas, for one."

Jonas unlatched the gate, and he and Gregor walked through together. They stood there companionably, Jonas looking down and smiling at the boy. Even TopGun seemed aware that they were about to part, for he licked at Gregor's hand.

"If you settled in Southampton, you'd be close to Portsmouth when his ship came in."

"But the Harrier pilots fly off before the ship docks."

"You can work those details out between you. And from the practical standpoint, didn't you win that contract on the aircraft carriers? If so, Southampton is a perfect location."

"The shipyard is on the River Tyne."

"So it is. Then Southampton is not quite perfect."

Not half as perfect as here, Sydney thought. *Here I could be happy with the sound of the birds singing, with early autumn flowers budding and trees shading the footpaths down to the river.* How often at home she had watched the river and wondered where it led and felt now that it had led to the Windrush.

"You did win that contract?" Abigail asked again.

"Phase one. Now Barrington is invited to submit blueprints. We have months of work ahead. Designing. Detailing. Coming up with a bid. So I—I have to get back to America."

"And after that?"

"After that," she said excitedly, "once we turn in the best blueprints—and we will beat our competitors—we will win the job. I expect to win, Abigail."

"You sound like Aaron Barrington did when he built his empire for himself."

"What he did, he did for Mother and me."

"What he did was leave his dreams for you to fulfill. I understand that now. I wanted someone to take up my work, to carry on my work with the children. I know now that we can only fulfill our own calling. Except for Millicent I used to wonder whether your father thought of anything but making a profit."

"He loved working. Loved proving himself."

266

"I'm afraid you are too much like him." She glanced toward Jonas. "I don't know whether anything can come for you and Jonas. I would like it to. But I can't make any promises. Don't leave unless you are certain that you must do so."

Abby caught Jonas's eye and waved. He waved back, smiling. *The same smile.* Still grinning, he leaned down and whispered in Gregor's ear. Gregor broke into a run toward the house as Jonas veered off toward the cottage, TopGun at his heels.

"Abigail, how can I know for certain?"

"Only you will know the answer to that. But don't miss out on happiness, Sydney. Don't let your father's death rob you of your own place in life. You're an intelligent woman; you could choose someone else to be CEO, if necessary. This Randolph for one."

Sydney felt herself flush, her anger rising in behalf of her father, in opposition to Randolph taking over. But Gregor bounded up the steps, cutting off any sharp comeback.

He came to a running stop by Abigail's chair. She cupped his chin and wiped a dirt smudge from his cheek. "You'd better go wash for supper."

He lingered. "You coming?"

"In a few minutes," she assured him.

He sent a shy glance toward Sydney. "Jonas is coming to supper. He'll be here in thirty minutes. Is that okay?"

"Of course," Abigail told him.

"But I get to sit by Jonas."

"He has two sides," Abigail said good-naturedly. "Now run along and tell Griselda to set another place at the table."

With the boy gone, something besides the southwesterly breeze stirred between them. Sydney felt uneasy at the thought of leaving this magical world and going back to her father's world. Her father's dreams. But something troubled her even more. Abigail Broderick and Jonas Willoughby might not be here when she came back.

Twenty-five

As Sydney and Abigail waited for Jonas to come back, they were caught in the timelessness of the never-ending beauty around them. The rolling limestone hills were rich with wildflowers, dotted with sheep grazing on grassy knolls, and ridged here and there with a goat path winding up from the valley. Early touches of autumn had already speckled the higher slopes in copper and burnt orange. Below them, the Windrush flowed lazily beneath the bridges, past a bank overhung with alders and cottonwoods and weeping willows.

"I heard you go out before dawn this morning, Sydney."

"I tried to tiptoe by your room. I ran into Reverend Rainford-Simms down by the Windrush. We sat on the riverbank and watched the burst of dawn reflecting on the water."

"Charles is comforting to be with. At least I find him so."

"He plans to come by this evening with communion for you and the Admiral." Sydney paused. "We talked about you and Jonas. About how close you are and how much alike you are."

"And did you find the answers you were looking for?"

"Some, but the more we talked, the more questions arose."

"You know, don't you?" Abigail asked calmly.

Sydney focused to where the tower of St. Michael's jutted toward the clouds. Clusters of buff-colored cottages lay on the sloping hillsides, their drystone walls overgrown with primrose climbers. She said at last, "Jonas is *your* son, isn't he?"

"Yes."

Sydney faced her. If she had expected to threaten Abigail with her past, she had misjudged the strength of the woman beside her. Abigail's smile, when it came, was composed, a smile so much like Jonas's. Warm. Friendly. She had obviously come to terms with whatever agony had haunted her over the years. In spite of the lingering pallor, hers was not a face of old age, but one of lasting beauty.

"How long have you known?" Abigail's voice held amazing calm. "Was it something I said—or did that gave me away?"

"It was the way you always look at Jonas—with such love. Does he know, Abigail?"

"No."

"Then you must tell him. You've waited far too long."

"It is because I waited that it's too late to tell him."

"I don't agree with you. He has a right to know."

"Dear child, in the maternity clinic where he was born, Lady Willoughby admitted me under her name. Lady Willoughby's name is on the birth certificate, and Lady Willoughby chose to take that secret to the grave. For Jonas's sake—not Lady Willoughby's—I kept my silence. A scandal now could still ruin his career."

"But the Admiral? The doctor who delivered him? Surely they know? Surely Sir James knows that Jonas isn't his son."

"But Jonas *is* his son."

Sydney gasped. "You mean—you and the Admiral?"

"Put that way, it sounds crude, scandalous. I must tell you, it took a long time for me to find my way back to peace. I have known God's love for forty years, but only since Charles came to Stow-on-the-Woodland have I fully comprehended God's forgiveness—and how to forgive myself as well."

Sydney thought of her own relationship with Randolph Iverson, the miserable blunders she had made. Forgiveness? Yes, it had made a difference in Abigail Broderick's life. But what price silence had cost her. Her son didn't even know the truth.

Abigail interrupted Sydney's thoughts. "Poor Tobias. I think he wanted to believe that Lady Willoughby had borne him a son. I wanted to tell him. Threatened to tell him. I was still foolish enough to love him—to think that he loved me. But Lady Willoughby made it quite clear that if I told him I would never see Jonas again. And the scandal would have ruined the Admiral's career."

"Surely, the Admiral must have known?"

"There were times when I was certain that he did. Hoped that he knew. Prayed that he knew that I was the one who had borne him a son. He never acknowledged knowing. His reputation and career were too important to him. And the prestige of Lady Willoughby's family name and wealth could not be ignored."

"What a selfish man."

"No, a proud man who worked hard to reach the top. Sir James wanted a son. Doted on him from a distance. He chided Lady Willoughby for years for not bearing him a child."

"It sounds like all he wanted was someone to carry on his legacy and walk in his footsteps."

"Tobias made plans for Jonas to follow in his footsteps before he was born. A Navy career. A family tradition." Her voice wavered. "Lady Helen threatened to keep my child from me. That was more than I could bear. Even so, for the first three months of Jonas's life I was ostracized—until that day he was baptized at St. Michael's. I was there watching, and I knew then that I would not allow her to keep me from my son any longer."

"How did she pull it off? You were the one pregnant."

"Tobias was often gone for months at a time. In the Far East. Deployed one place or the other. Long absences from each other did not seem to trouble them. Or perhaps it only troubled Lady Willoughby. When he was at sea, Lady Willoughby often traveled abroad. And that's what we did. For the last six months of my pregnancy, we lived in the French countryside in a rented villa."

"I thought Jonas was born in this country."

"He was, Sydney. My pregnancy was complicated. I was in my forties—facing the birth of my first child. My only child," she said sadly. "I insisted that the Admiral's child be born on British soil. And so we came back to England to a small maternity clinic in the North country. I was quite ill by then and didn't know until afterwards that she had registered me in her name. And so my son was born and listed on the records as Helen's son."

She sighed. "When we left the clinic, Lady Willoughby carried the baby to the car. She drove into the next town, stopped the car, handed me some money, and told me that I was never to return to the manor again. Griselda guessed, of course. But she has always been the loyal one. Lady Willoughby rarely flew down to meet her husband when his ship came in, fearing another woman being there. But people here in Stow-on-the-Woodland thought of them as the beautiful young Helen, the dashing naval officer, the devoted couple."

"Why the facade of a happy marriage?"

"James bowed under the public image. He wanted nothing to mar his career. Poor James. The Admiral had waited long years to pick a bride and Helen was by far the most lovely to choose from. She owned the manor, had the social standing in London that appealed to him. Money was always on her side, but once she met the handsome naval officer, she determined to marry him."

She sighed. "Even though he was much older, the Admiral was the envy of her friends. They guessed even then that he would go far in his career. Helen wanted to go with him. He remained rakishly handsome at forty-six when Jonas was born and still charming to other women."

She choked up as she said, "Lady Willoughby loved him and felt convinced that if she bore a child for the Admiral, he would never look at another woman again. When she found out I was pregnant with her husband's child, she wanted to thrash me. And then she offered to protect my

271

reputation in the village where I had grown up; in exchange the child would be raised as her own."

"She was young—healthy. Why not have her own child?"

"She had been thrown from a horse as a young child and severely injured. Complications eventually led to a hysterectomy. But the Admiral didn't know that."

Sydney touched Abigail's arm. "If Lady Willoughby took this secret to her grave, why have you risked sharing it with me?"

"I have to trust someone. Who better than Millicent Barrington's daughter? I think you will do right by my son if I die before my will is revised." She rested for a moment. "My health has been failing for some time, my heart flabby and undependable. When I went into Edmund's office some months before my last heart attack, he made offers to buy the property from me. He had some scheme for opening up the village to tourism. I had gone to his father all my life. When Edmund took over his father's clients, I thought I could trust him."

As the sun lowered on the horizon, the glare blinded them. They adjusted their chairs, drawing back into the shade. Sydney slipped a sweater around Abigail's shoulders. "Mr. Gallagher may be unscrupulous enough to carry it off. I've met him. He does have an elaborate plan to turn Stow-on-the-Woodland commercial, but the village would lose its quaint charm. It's time for you to trust my friend Jeff. Let's get your will written the way you want it. We'll have Edmund meet you here."

Abigail began to fidget with the button on her sweater. "Just weeks before my heart attack, I called for another appointment. Again Edmund offered to buy me out. When I refused, he put me off. He said he had to bring in some papers from London. I begged him not to delay—to help me get my affairs in order at once. He promised we would draw up the papers the next time we met."

"You should have seen another lawyer."

"When I told him I would travel to London and consult with one of his partners, Edmund threatened to reveal things about the Admiral and Jonas. I fear he may know that Jonas is my son. How, I cannot tell you, but we reached a shouting match that set my heart to racing. He told me I was a fool to keep the property for Jonas. Jonas had no interest in it."

Her voice weakened. "I hung up on Edmund, but before I did, I told him that you would manage the property for Jonas. After all, you were my friend's daughter."

"You didn't even know me."

She closed her eyes for a moment. "But I wanted to trust you. My heart was just riding wild. I was desperate to right the wrong done so long ago."

"The wrong? Does that relate to the hold that you had over Lady Willoughby? Her property in exchange for your silence?"

"It was more than that, Sydney. With the property in my name, I could go on taking care of the children—and still be near Jonas. The Admiral wanted her to sell the property so they could move back to London. Tobias disliked the house filled with children when he came home. He had difficulty enough warming to his own son. I would have lost the right to care for the children. The right to see Jonas. So I went to Helen and threatened to tell the Admiral the truth. To tell him that Jonas was my son. I laid out my terms."

"What terms, Abigail?"

Her breathing seemed more rapid now, her eyes tired. "The property would go into my name for as long as I lived. At least one wing of the manor would always be kept for the children under my care. The Willoughbys would maintain the stables and the garden. And I would never be refused the right to see my son."

Abigail's lower lip had turned a bluish gray, but she went on. "The property was to go back to Helen at my death— I was so much older. And Helen would, of course, leave it to her son."

"And all that changed when Lady Willoughby died?"

"Yes," she whispered. "We must not speak of this again. But if I die before all of this is settled, promise me that you will make certain that Edmund Gallagher is not permitted to lay claim to Broadshire Manor. The land belongs to Jonas."

Abigail looked exhausted. "You have been good for me, Sydney. And if that friend of yours can help us . . ."

"I'll have Jeff make the arrangements for tomorrow."

She smiled. "If he doesn't come in time, the land is yours. I trust you to make certain that Jonas can lay claim to it." A smile lit her face. "There! Jonas is coming now."

The sight of him awakened Sydney's own senses, her longing to be needed, wanted by Commander Willoughby. His hair was still wet from the shower, his handsome face obviously just shaved. He was wearing tan slacks and a short-sleeve pullover shirt of blue chambray, a brilliant blue against his bronzed skin. Long-limbed and muscular, he strode briskly toward them. A confident, surefooted man. As he climbed the steps, the woody scent of his cologne was more pungent than the flowering shrub by the porch.

It was the same cologne he had been wearing that night by the Windrush. His charm—the details of that night surged back and forth in her mind like the rushes at the water's edge. She recalled the mesmerizing effect of his deep-set eyes meeting hers. Of admitting to him that she was cold in her bareback dress and having his arm slip around her, his soft cardigan sweater touch her bare back. She heard the thumping beat of his heart as he held her. Felt the strength of his arm and muscular body and was ready for the intensity of his warm lips as they sought hers.

But what had that moment at the Windrush meant to Jonas? She forced herself to look at Jonas now and traced his strong profile in her mind's eye. Saw again that stubborn jaw so much like the Admiral's.

He glanced at Abigail and in his deep, hypnotic voice said, "We'd better get you inside before the midges eat you alive."

His eyes were on Abigail, yet Sydney felt certain that he was simply biding his time, pacing himself, waiting for just the right moment to turn his attention her way.

He held Abigail's hand and helped her to her feet. Then he tucked her arm in his, leaving Sydney to follow behind them. And still Sydney felt certain that his own need of her had awakened the moment he found them sitting by the fountain.

They were into the main hallway before he turned back to her and smiled. "I was wondering, Syd, are you busy after supper?"

Her words jumbled in her throat. "I. Well, I usually—"

Abigail glanced back. "Of course, she's free. I am well enough to put myself to bed and strong enough to at least read to the children until Griselda is ready to bathe them."

"What did you have in mind, Jonas?" Sydney asked shyly.

"Veronica's Tea Shoppe is closed by seven, so I thought we could walk down to Chutman's Pub."

"Isn't the pub for men only?"

"Not here in Stow-on-the-Woodland. It's a community affair where people gather to talk and drink."

"I don't drink."

"Not even tea?" he teased. "And they serve their bread-and-butter pudding, hot and creamy. We could skip supper here and have a light meal at the pub."

"No," Abigail warned. "Gregor is counting on sitting beside you at the table. You must not disappoint him."

"Oh, in the excitement I forgot."

He put his arm around Abigail, around his own mother without knowing, and moved down the corridor toward Griselda's kitchen. But Sydney felt contentment. She would be with Jonas this evening. Out on their own. Walking the footpath to the pub and the Windrush with no one else with them. She looked again at his strong arm resting so gently on Abigail's shoulder and thought with the pounding of her own heart, and a flush of her cheeks, *tonight, perhaps, his arm will be around me.*

Twenty-six

Abigail did not sleep after supper but rested in the comfort of her own room with its thick lace curtains on the windows and elegant seventeenth-century tapestry on the wall. Griselda had lit a fire in the fireplace and the crackling of burning logs added to the coziness. Keeley and Tesa sat at the quaint desk with its pigeonholes stuffed with their drawings, each girl laboriously sketching a picture of Keeley's Shetland pony.

Gregor poked his head in the door. "Miss Abigail, I want to go down to Chutman's Pub with Jonas."

"You've just had supper."

"I won't eat much."

"But Jonas is taking Sydney out for the evening."

His face shadowed. "They said I could come."

"You invited yourself?"

He refused to meet her eyes. His toes turned in, the way they did when he was making excuses. Her heart went out to him. "Gregor, give them some time alone."

"She hangs around him all the time."

Go gently with him, Abigail told herself. "Stay with me this evening. We haven't had a good visit for a long time."

"If you don't let me go, I can't catch up with them."

So he would be the uninvited guest. Firmly she said, "You are not to go this time. Try to understand." His dark eyes blazed as she said, "Why not work on one of your model planes in here? You could stay up until I retire."

"Jonas is helping me with the plane."

Jonas again. "Then let me rest a bit. After that we'll pay the Admiral a visit. Sir James likes it when you call on him."

"I saw him today. He was reading his *Navy News* and said Jonas's aircraft carrier is docking in Portsmouth soon."

"Gregor, was he reading or just looking at the pictures?"

"He tried to make out the words himself. Sometimes Sydney reads to him when I can't. She does everything for the Admiral that I used to do. I wish she'd go home again."

"Jonas would feel bad if she went away."

He kicked the door, his boyish face anguished. "I know."

"Come here, Gregor. Jonas doesn't love you any less. He just wants to be with Sydney sometimes."

"I think he wants to marry her, and then he'll go away. I heard him tell the Reverend Rainford-Simms—"

"You followed Jonas down there? Were you eavesdropping?"

As he reached her bedside, she cupped his sun-scaled cheeks. "Gregor, Griselda and I will be here for you even if Jonas and Sydney get married."

"He'll send me off to Gordonstoun just to get rid of me."

"No, not to get rid of you. He's proud of you—like a son. He wants you to go there because it was his boarding school."

His lip quivered. "Do I have to go, Miss Abigail?"

"I thought you wanted to go. You'd meet so many boys your age. And have the chance to play so many sports."

"I'm not good in sports."

"Oh, but you run faster than anyone I know. And you are getting better in soccer."

"I might never come back to the manor."

"Of course, you will." She had been too quick with her answer. He was still a little boy who needed her. "Would you rather go to the primary school here at Stow-on-the-Woodland?"

She tousled his hair. He smelled of shampoo, his breath minty from toothpaste. Sydney must have hugged him, for his shirt held the faint fragrance of her French perfume.

"I'll talk to Jonas," she said. "He wants to take you up to Gordonstoun for a visit. You will go, won't you? He'd be disappointed."

"He won't get in the car and go away without me?"

Everyone he had known in Kosovo had left him. "Jonas would never do that. I love you, Gregor. So does Jonas."

He nestled against her arm. "Are you going to leave us?"

"I don't want to, but I'm ill. Someday I'll have to go away, but I'll go on loving you. I just won't be here like I am now."

He seemed to understand. Seemed to accept. Gregor and the O'Reillys would be the last of her hidden children. The circle was closing in, the retreat from Dunkirk coming to a final close. Abigail Broderick at seventeen had been free-spirited, absolutely certain that she would live forever. But on the march to the burning city of Dunkirk, she had feared not living at all. Now she did not fear death, but where had the decades gone?

Was she really seventy-seven? Inside, she was still free-spirited; outside, dignified. Serene. She knew as she slipped her arm around Gregor's bony shoulders that her work was almost over. No one would pick up her dreams and run with them. The course she had run was her own. She wanted only to hear a "well done" when she reached the end of her journey.

Abigail kissed the top of Gregor's head. She wanted more than anything to be there for him as he grew up, to help him over the pitfalls, to perhaps go with him when he saw his own country again, but she knew she would not live long enough to do so.

"I want to rest now, Gregor. Would you take the girls down to Griselda? It's almost their bedtime."

He went obediently to the desk and folded Tesa's drawing book and lowered the rolltop. Tesa slipped off her chair and ran and flung herself at Abigail. Keeley stood shyly watching them.

"Sleep well, little ones. And count the sheep the minute your heads hit the pillow."

"I am done with counting sheep," Keeley announced. "Sydney told me I can count jasmine and roses instead."

She smiled. "Then tomorrow tell me how many you counted."

The door closed behind them. She lay against her pillows, listening to their voices as they walked down the hall. When their steps faded, the ringing of the bell at St. Michael's awakened her memories. She caught the scent of flowers outside her window and shut her eyes to search for sheep and jasmine and roses to count. The movie of her past was already in play, the reel spinning. Spinning a seventeen-year-old back to the long line of soldiers standing on the sands of Dunkirk. They stood there, shading their eyes, looking out on the choppy waters waiting for ships to rescue them.

And her hidden past played before her, bringing with it both joy and sadness. She remembered the coldness of the soldier's helmet on her head. But the face that she saw was not her own. It was Sydney in the British uniform looking up at Neil Irwin and asking, "Why didn't you marry Abigail?"

Neil's cheerful voice echoed in her memory. "Ah, mate, I'd have married my sweetheart after the war. But the battle of Normandy came along."

The reel kept spinning. Hermann and Isaac with grown-up faces, dressed in khaki undershirts and clinging to a dinghy. The long line of children who had come to her. Santos. Conon. Tyler. Rebecca.

The reel jammed, then started again. Herself—a woman in her thirties with rusty brown hair timidly gripping the knocker at the manor and looking up at a tall naval officer with smashing good looks. The beaches of Dunkirk were lost in a mist, and she was walking to the top of the golden hills in the Cotswolds, laughing up at the officer with the rakish smile. The dreadful realization that she was pregnant, the sin that almost destroyed her. But Charles Rainford-

Simms had come to St. Michael's with his ministry of love and forgiveness.

The kaleidoscope of a lifetime. The changing patterns of her life. Dappled rainbows, checkered, twisted turns that had brought her to this moment. She saw the young Abigail Broderick. Saw the old Abigail. Watched herself go from rusty brown hair to silvery gray. Her dreams and destiny all one now. Woven into the pattern, she saw herself fleeing to the continent to Lady Willoughby's private French villa. Saw her body distorted with pregnancy and the beautiful Lady Willoughby planning for Abigail's child as though the baby had formed in her own womb. And the plan conceived that made the child forever a Willoughby.

There was no real sleep, only the drifting of the yesterdays in her memory. A pregnancy wrought with difficulties. A maternity clinic in the north country. The reel of deception kept spinning. Jonas's birth recorded as Lady Willoughby's child. The nun wiring the Admiral that a son had been born. Then leaving the clinic on that sunless day and being told she was no longer needed. Ever.

The end of the reel spun off. Her return to the manor months later, refusing to be separated from her son another day. The threat to tell the truth. The Admiral had stared at the child in Abigail's arms. For a moment it seemed like he knew, but he said nothing. Even now, Abigail saw Lady Willoughby thrusting the contract into the Admiral's hands. Saw the sadness in his eyes. "Abigail wants the manor. She wants to go on taking in children."

He had glanced at Abigail. "Let her have anything, Helen."

The anguished voice of Helen: "You know, don't you, James?"

The cold, noncommittal "Know what, my dear Helen?"

"That you would lose everything if she told the truth." Helen had touched his cheek, having always loved him. "So, James, what you cannot openly admit, you cannot deny."

They signed, and Abigail, still holding Jonas, had said, "It will go no further. Ever. You can have your ships and Lady Willoughby this child. But I must watch him grow up."

Abigail's life had been capricious. Stimulating. Painful. Convoluted. Happy. Ever moving her forward. The many images all there. But even here in this room she was covered by an arc of forgiveness. It had all been part of growing up, growing old. The beginning tying in with the end. So dying was just a part of living, the capstone more glorious than the golden hills.

She was about to sew that last stitch on the unfinished quilt of her life. Was she to bury her secrets as Lady Willoughby had done? Was she to leave no visible legacy of love for Jonas? Abigail felt the heart flutter that came at unexpected moments. The lamps in her room formed shadows on the wall, highlighting the colors in the tapestry. She had one small hope. If her own courage failed her, then one day—and Sydney would know the right time—Sydney Barrington would tell Jonas the whole truth.

Twenty-seven

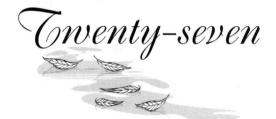

The next morning Sydney sat alone on the top of the knoll. The happy cries of the children and the lamenting notes of Jonas's bagpipes wafted back toward her. As she thought of the pleasant evening at the pub with Jonas—of his strong arm around her, a shadow fell across her path.

She glanced up into the gaunt face of a stranger, a man younger than Jonas. If his cheeks were fuller, his skin less gray, she would have thought him attractive.

"You sent word that you wanted to see me," he said.

"And I'm surprised that you came. Sit down, please."

He held his ribs and eased down on the ground beside her. He took the apple she offered and bit into it. "Are my children living with you now?" he asked.

His accent was decidedly Irish, and she knew for certain that this was Keeley's father—the terrorist that she was supposed to fear. "We're all staying up at the manor."

"How are they, Miss Barrington?"

So Charles has told him my name. "All six of them are down there with Jonas Willoughby."

He winced at the name. "Yes. Who else but Jonas would be playing the bagpipes? Is he good to the Irish children as well?"

"He tries to be. Danny adores Mrs. Quigley."

"All of the children end up liking her. And Keeley?"

She turned and looked into his haunted eyes and pitied him. "She misses her father. Prays every night that he will come back. We've become good friends and often go riding together."

"I've seen you riding out on the hills. She seems happy with you. Take my children to America with you."

She laughed. "They have no passports."

His hand fell limply to his side. He had lost interest in the apple. Or perhaps he was too sick to even chew it. "I'll write a letter—giving you permission to take them. Will you?"

He was handing her the responsibility of his children. Had she come all the way to England for this stranger in his brooding silence to ask her help? Even on the open hillside, the odor of his festering wounds was strong.

"Do you want to stay and see the children?"

His cold pale eyes softened as he rubbed his whiskery chin. "I won't put them through another good-bye."

He began to cough, a violent spasm that left fresh spots of blood on his shirt. She reached out and touched his arm. "You're bleeding. I could send Dr. Wallis. You need medical attention."

"A friend is looking after me, Miss Barrington."

"Then go before Jonas and the children come back."

"Will you tell Jonas where I am?"

"I don't know for certain where you're staying. I'd only be guessing. And—you haven't told me your name."

His smile twisted the gaunt lines in his face. "Which one of us are you protecting?"

He jerked to his feet. More drops of blood fell on the ground where he had been sitting. Far below, the lamenting wail of the bagpipes ceased. The children began racing up the hillside. Keeley stopped. Looked. And ran harder.

"You can barely stand. Let me help you?" Sydney offered.

He shook his head. "Someone is waiting for me."

"Next Sunday, I'll leave pictures of the children at the baptismal font. One of Keeley on her pony. One of both of them."

"I'll find them there. Thank you."

"Go," she said. "The children are coming."

Conon coughed as he slipped into the woods. And then the sound of him, the sight of him, disappeared.

Keeley stumbled into Sydney's arms. "Where did my papa go?" She pounded against Sydney's chest. "Where did he go?"

"I don't know for certain, Keeley."

Dear God, forgive me, she thought. *But Conon is right. He is too sick for them to see him this way.*

Keeley's sobs subsided as Sydney held her. "He didn't even wave."

"Maybe you just wanted it to be him, honey."

Jonas dragged up the hill with the other children clinging to him. "What's wrong with her?" he asked, bewildered.

"She misses her father."

Jonas knelt on one knee and pointed to his back. "Hop on. It's your turn for a free pony ride, Keeley."

"You're not my pony."

"I'm a make-believe one."

Shyly she climbed on his back, the other children standing around with envy in their eyes. Jonas supported her chubby legs. Keeley locked her arms around his neck. He shrugged her more securely on his back and then looked at Sydney with a penetrating gaze. "I won't ask any questions. We agreed to trust each other."

"I know. Thank you."

"Sydney, tomorrow we're going on a picnic of our own. Just the two of us. The children aren't invited."

Gregor scowled. "No children," Jonas said, silencing his objection. "What do you say, Miss Barrington? Veronica at the tea shop promised to pack us a picnic box."

"I'd love to go with you. Just the two of us."

He went galloping off with Keeley clinging to him. Sydney covered Conon's drops of blood with her shoe. She felt grateful to Jonas for not asking questions that she could not answer. She had wanted to meet with Conon O'Reilly. *She had met with a stranger.*

Gregor slipped his hand in hers. "Don't look so sad, Sydney. You're the one going on a picnic with Jonas tomorrow."

"I know." She felt a lightness kick in, a momentary happiness that brought color to her cheeks, joy to her heart.

Sydney took the items of food from Veronica's basket as Jonas stretched contentedly on his back on the picnic rug. He peeked at her. "I'd like this time together to go on forever."

She pressed his hand against her cheek. "It can't. I have to go home. I have a company to run and they can't do the job without me."

"What a high-powered operative you are. Buying shipyards. Building carriers."

"That's not fair. I didn't ask to be the head of Dad's company when he died. I stumbled into that position, but I'm telling you, I conquered it with the Barrington spirit."

"Then why did you come to the Cotswolds if you were only going to turn around and leave me?"

"I think I came looking for a special place—a special person—and I found them both here."

The waters of the Windrush bubbled a few feet from them. "Jonas, I love being near water—listening to the sound of a waterfall or watching a river like this one coursing around the countryside." He laughed up at her, but she still said, "It's always the same—the sound of water makes me peaceful."

"I feel the same way. That's why I like going to sea."

"It's strange. Both sets of my parents died in water, and yet I still find the sound of water peaceful."

He reached across the picnic rug and took her hand in his again. "Not strange at all. Water is symbolic of life. It keeps flowing endlessly. What I regret most is how untroubled I was when my ship was deployed to another crisis point. The Navy and going to sea was my life. I expected Louise to understand."

"Maybe you expected too much."

As Sydney took the rest of Veronica's surprises from the basket, she saw Lucas striding toward them with a young couple. The girl was short and pudgy with a pretty smiling face, the young man lean and whistling as he approached.

He winked at Sydney and gave Jonas a nudge with his boot. "On your feet, man. You have guests."

At the sound of his friend's voice, Jonas rolled to his side and scrambled to his feet. They pounded each other.

"Jock."

"Commander." Jock glanced at Sydney. "I see we can finally stop our search for a London debutante."

"Sydney, this is Joseph Hollinsworth and his wife, Kathleen. Only we call him Jock." He pounded his friend's arm again. "I thought you'd be back on the carrier by now."

"I'm back with the squadron at Morayshire. We're expecting to be posted to the *Invincible* the next time she comes into port. But it won't be the same flying wingman for someone else."

Kathleen said shyly, "You're not flying wingman this time, Jock. If you don't tell Jonas, I will." Proudly, she said, "They've promoted Jock to squadron commander."

A cloud washed over Jonas's face, but he was quick to recover. "Getting liberal with their promotions, aren't they?"

"Desperate. You know I'd step aside if you were going back."

"Someday, Jock. What about you two joining us? Veronica packed plenty of food. What do you say, Sydney?"

"That Veronica thought we'd stay here for a week."

Jonas gave her a quick wink. "Don't I wish."

Jock dropped down beside them. "Jonas, I've been doing weekend flights in my uncle's Learjet while I'm waiting for the *Invincible* to come back. I solo now. So I can take her up alone."

He chuckled. "My uncle's business is booming, particularly in the Scandinavian countries. We flew in here today—and my uncle is off to Finland, flying commercial. We have a flight scheduled next weekend. I'll meet my uncle in Helsinki. Head to Stockholm to pick up some passengers and back to London. If you're free, you could go along."

"Some other time, Jock." He seemed suddenly aware that Lucas was still hovering around. "No need for you to stand by, Lucas. My friends and I have a lot of visiting to do."

As Lucas stomped off, Sydney handed a plate to Kathleen. "What will you do now that your husband is going back to sea?"

"I'll be in London with my parents waiting for his return."

Is that how it was? Waiting for a return, even before the ship left the harbor? Was that the kind of life she would have with Jonas Willoughby? A life where she would feel like an intruder on his time? But Kathleen was bubbling with joy, still flirting with Jock as though they had just married.

Between bites, Jonas teased, "Jock, did you reach the goals you set for your leave?"

Jock slipped his arm around his wife. "If you count Kathleen being sick to her stomach every morning—and sending me out at midnight for pickles just to get in practice when the obsession strikes her, everything went well."

Kathleen blushed. "But I never liked pickles," she admitted, taking a bite from the one that Sydney offered her.

Jock patted his wife's stomach. "This is my reason for taking on my uncle's jobs. Kathleen has a doctor's appointment in London next week. And," he said, "we might as well put in the request now. Jonas, we're going to want you to stand up with us when we have the baby christened."

He stole a fresh glimpse toward Sydney. "And if you stay on board, you're invited too."

287

Sydney and Jonas fell into an awkward silence. "Look," Jock apologized. "We're not rushing you. We just thought— well, we thought you had something going here between you. Sorry."

On Tuesday, as Edmund Gallagher knocked on the old oak door at the manor, Jeff VanBurien climbed the steps behind him. Edmund acknowledged the American with a curt nod and stepped into the great hall at Griselda's invitation.

"Mrs. Quigley, I have an appointment with Miss Broderick. Would you be so good as to tell her I've arrived?"

"Same thing," VanBurien said cheerily. "I have an appointment with Miss Broderick as well."

Griselda wiped her hands on her apron. "She's expecting you both. She's in the library waiting."

Edmund stalled. He glared at Jeff. "She sent for me regarding personal matters. I am her solicitor. So if you would be so good as to wait your turn—"

Griselda said, "She expects you both at the same time. She's in the library and doesn't like to be kept waiting."

Jeff extended his hand. "After you, Mr. Gallagher."

Edmund had just stepped into the massive library when he saw Sydney. The angry curve of his mouth tightened. He crunched his jaw, the crackling audible across the room. "So Dr. Wallis was right, Miss Barrington. You have settled in at Broadshire Manor."

Abigail sat with great dignity behind the Admiral's massive desk. She was wearing a blue velvet dress with a high collar that had always looked striking on her. Yet this morning the neckline seemed too big. She was indeed ill. Losing weight.

"Gentlemen," she said, and her voice was as strong as it had ever been, "we were getting worried that you might be late."

Jeff grinned. "I believe we're right on time, ma'am."

Edmund's annoyance blew out of control. "Abigail, I believe you made an appointment with me. I have other clients at the office. Can we get on with this?"

"Of course. But I have appointments with all of you. I believe you and Mr. VanBurien have met under different circumstances? And this is a dear friend of mine. Sydney Barrington." The smile lines at Abigail's eyes deepened. "Sydney, this is the solicitor I was telling you about. Edmund Gallagher."

"We've met," Sydney said coolly. "I believe he was urging me to sell the manor when I thought I was inheriting this place."

Edmund continued to bluff his way. "We have business to discuss, Abigail. Perhaps your friends could leave us alone?"

"No. As you know, Miss Barrington is presently my sole heir. You can understand her concern that her personal lawyer be present to defend her rights."

Jeff casually pulled up a chair and sat beside Sydney.

Abigail flashed them a warm smile. "Mr. VanBurien and Sydney both know that I intend to change my will today. Edmund, if you refuse to cooperate, then Mr. VanBurien will arrange for one of your partners to journey here from London. Is that understood?"

Edmund's mouth grew taut, stretching his lips to a narrow line. He was tasting humiliation and he knew it—facing defeat and knew it. He cast a glance around the magnificent room and knew that his dream of ownership had slipped away.

"Is there a problem, Edmund?"

Sweat drenched his shirt. "Of course not."

"Then perhaps we should get started?"

Wallis had warned him. He had gone too far. Word would spread quickly through the village. He panicked, wondering how he could replace the funds he had misappropriated at the London office.

Edmund sank into the chair, the meeting already out of his hands, the taste of gall in his mouth.

Sydney left the library three hours later with a splitting headache. She had not enjoyed seeing Edmund Gallagher go down in defeat. The errors that he had made in Abigail's business matters had been pointed out and the legal implications spelled out by Jeff in a language that Edmund understood. In the end, Abigail insisted on a simple, handwritten will; and when it was done, Jeff and Sydney penned their names as witnesses. Sydney came from the room, no longer the heir to 250 acres of land and six children, but she shared Abigail's joy. The Willoughby property would pass from generation to generation as it had always done.

Sydney headed toward her room, but Griselda stopped her. "Hurry, Sydney. That young man from America is on the phone."

Randolph again, she thought. How many times had he called since her arrival in England? Hadn't the day been bad enough? She built a fist around the receiver and said, "Hello. Sydney Barrington speaking."

"Syd, it's Randolph. When are you coming home? I miss you."

"I don't know."

"You don't know when you're coming or whether I miss you?"

"A little bit of both."

"It's that Navy commander, isn't it? He's answered the phone several times when I called. Thinks I'm your business partner."

"You are."

"I should hate the guy. Whenever I ask him where you are, he says you're with the children or Abigail Broderick. You're different somehow, Sydney. In your letters, you seem happier than you've ever been."

"I *am* happier."

"When are you coming home?"

"You don't like the way I run things when I am there."

"I worry about the way you rush into big decisions. You're still trying to salvage Aaron's folly, and now Daron Emery tells me you've bid on another shipyard in Italy."

"Some of the European designers are so far ahead of us. We're in global competition. Remember?" She heard the competitive spirit in her own words.

"The only competition I'm worried about is that Navy commander. If you think the Europeans are so far advanced, maybe you'd better think about living abroad permanently."

She heard the bite in his words and felt defensive. "If I thought it meant taking Barrington straight to the top, then I would make this my permanent residence."

Or, she thought reflectively, *if it means finding my castle in the air—my happiness, then, yes, I will change my address.*

"Don't do that. I'd miss you."

"You sound like I've already made the decision to stay."

"I think you have in your heart. Do you know what you will do with the house and the cabin?"

"Now you have my house up for sale! Those are things I would have to work out. But I think I want to keep the cabin. I want Keeley and Danny—"

"The kids?"

"Yes, I want them to spend some of their summers there. I loved that place. I want them to love it too."

"You've changed, Sydney. Aaron's lost his hold on you."

"No, I've just found something I want more than Aaron's kingdom."

Twenty-eight

The morning after the meeting with Gallagher, Sydney left for an emergency meeting at the Jarrow Shipyard. On returning days later she found the cottage closed and Jonas gone. Gregor was gone too, and a black-and-white collie was spending most of her time beside the Admiral's bed.

It was lonely at the manor without them, but on Friday Sydney put on a cheerful face as she walked into a kitchen filled with the fragrant aroma of fresh baking. "Smells good in here, Mrs. Quigley."

Griselda beamed. "So you're awake, Sydney. There's a fresh pot of tea, and I will have something hot from the oven soon."

"Any word from Jonas? They've been gone a week. I thought they'd be home by now."

"Did you now?" Her eyes twinkled. "After Gordonstoun, he planned to take the boy to Morayshire to visit his old squadron."

"But I thought Jonas was taking me on that trip—at least that's what he told me."

"Guess he changed his mind—what with you off to that shipyard of yours without telling him."

"I left so early I didn't want to wake him."

"No matter. It's best this way. Gave Gregor a chance to have Jonas to himself. But Jonas practically has the boy signed up for the Navy and flying a Sea Harrier."

"I hope he won't pressure him about boarding school."

"Abigail won't let Jonas do that. Gregor is her boy. And she thinks he'll do best with another year or two at the village school. Jonas is like his father. Once he makes up his mind there's no stopping him. He wants Gregor to have the best preparation for going with the Royal Navy."

"Gregor is only nine."

"Jonas went away long before that. He went from his trainers into training for the Navy. And when he bid for flight school, I thought the Admiral would have a stroke."

"But the Admiral wanted his son in the Navy."

"Commanding a ship, not crashing on some flight deck."

It would never work out, Sydney thought. *A little boy and the Navy are stiff competition.* Yet, she would gladly have gone to Gordonstoun and Scotland with them—to fill in those missing pieces of Jonas's life and to meet his Uncle Ian.

Sydney filled her cup as Griselda said, "Lucas was just here asking for you. He found your riding stick. It's over there." She nodded toward the table. "Said he kept meaning to give it back. Thought you might need it the next time you go riding."

It felt as if Griselda had punched her in the stomach. Sydney gripped the table and sat down, the cup rattling in the saucer as she put it on the table. "Did Lucas say anything else?"

"Just that you should be more careful next time. It upsets him if anything gets out of place in the stables. He doesn't like much, but he does like keeping a watchful eye on those horses. Those stallions are probably the only friends he has."

"You don't think much of Lucas, do you?"

"What's there to like?"

"He's good to the Admiral."

"It works best when he stays in the west wing and I stay in the kitchen. Don't go getting yourself in trouble, Sydney. Not with Lucas. He's a private man. He doesn't like people overstepping their limits in the stables."

"I never intended to." She ran her finger moodily around the edge of her cup. "I'll be more careful next time I go riding. It's just—oh, never mind."

Mrs. Quigley turned from the old iron oven, mopping her brow. "Are you wanting to tell Griselda all about it?"

"I should talk to Jonas first. I just hope I'm here long enough to do so."

"You won't be if that young man of yours has his way. He called again this morning."

"Randolph called again? Was anything wrong?"

"Same thing today and yesterday and the day before and last week. The only thing wrong is he wants you back there to marry him. Usually Mr. Iverson just leaves a message for you. Takes care to spell his name one letter at a time, like as though I couldn't hear him. But this morning he told me to make it clear to you that he'll fly over here if you don't go home."

"He would. But Randolph is right. Daron Emery is doing a splendid job at Jarrow Shipyard. And Abigail is getting better. So I have no excuse to stay any longer."

Griselda's thick brows puckered. "None of us want you to go." Her voice cracked. She sniffed against her flour-white wrist. "Even the Admiral thinks you're part of the crew."

"I'm beginning to leave dust marks on the welcome mat." She met Griselda's steady gaze. "I hoped Jonas would get back so I could tell him good-bye."

The twinkle was back. "I thought you'd be more observant than that. He came back late last night."

Hot humiliation burned Sydney's cheeks. "Is he avoiding me?"

"Ask him," she called over her shoulder. "Poor boy doesn't know his own mind. And Gregor is certainly not going to volunteer the information. I can tell by your voice that you didn't know."

"I haven't seen Jonas since the picnic."

"That was more than a week ago. And he was upset when he didn't find you here for breakfast the morning you left for the shipyard."

"Didn't you tell him where I went?"

"Wasn't my job to tell him. That's between the two of you. Once you took off to that shipyard of yours, he moped around. I need to warn you. I think Jonas is trying to sort out his feelings about you, and you're not making it easy." She put her hands on her hips, a pack of wisdom wrapped behind her gruff manner. "Sydney, you are going to rub the design off that cup, so stop playing with it and get yourself another cup of tea."

"Would you like me to help you bake?" Sydney offered.

"Beautiful morning like this and you have nothing to do except help me in the kitchen? The children are with Abigail. So go for a horseback ride. Enjoy yourself."

"I don't want to face Lucas right now. Not alone."

Mrs. Quigley mulled that one over with her arms deep in flour, forming dumplings and breakfast rolls. "Such problems you have. You could help Boris in the garden."

"I'd rather help Jonas." The words slipped out before she could retrieve them. "I don't know what made me say that."

"That's the trouble. You don't know your own heart." She took the loaves of nut bread from the oven, the aroma permeating the kitchen. Sydney's mouth watered.

"Now me, for instance—" Mrs. Quigley fanned her flushed face with the muslin cloth that served as her apron. "I knew right off with my husband, Arthur."

"You never talk about him."

"Can't without getting all choked up. I met him out there on the hills tending sheep for his uncle. Arthur was much like Jonas. Strong and tall, and a right handsome one. We were both young—me, I was just sixteen. I knew right off, once he showed up at Chutman's Pub. I chased him from the day I met him. Married him just past my eighteenth birthday. We settled here in Stow-on-the-Woodland so Arthur could farm the land."

"What happened to him?"

"Died with consumption—eight years after we married. Abby was my lifeline, what with me losing my Arthur like that."

"You should have married again."

The tired lines around Mrs. Quigley's eyes softened. "There can be only one Arthur in a lifetime."

There could be only one Jonas in a lifetime.

"Abby talked the Willoughbys into hiring me. When Lady Willoughby died, I stayed on. Wouldn't have 'cepting my friend Abigail was living at the manor by then. Even then, I thought I wouldn't stay on—not with the Admiral fussing like he did whenever he came home on leave and saw all them children."

"You're good with the children. That's what makes you and Abigail both so special."

Griselda set another baking pan in the oven and reset her timer. For a second Sydney thought Griselda's shoulders quivered. "Griselda, if I said something wrong, I'm sorry."

She snorted. "You'll be more sorry if you let Jonas go."

Sydney's cheeks burned. "I don't know what you mean."

Their eyes met again. "Been here all these weeks and don't know what I mean? Every time you look at him you go scarlet."

Sydney put her hands to her cheeks to hide the burning. "I guess it's like you and Arthur—I've never known anyone like Jonas."

"Then go down to his cottage and tell him. Can't hurt. Might help. I did a bit of rushing after Arthur, once I met him."

"Gregor will be down at the cottage."

"Not this morning. This morning the children are with Abigail, and after that, Gregor promised me he would take the Admiral's noon meal to him. That means standing by and making certain the Admiral eats something. Since Gregor usually comes back with an empty tray, I figure he is doing most of the eating. But that boy understands the Admiral. Likes him. It's good for the children to have responsibility. Good for Gregor to be needed."

Sydney ran her finger around the rim of her cup again. "Griselda, you're deliberately keeping Gregor busy."

"I most certainly am. He's had Jonas to himself for a whole week. I didn't bake all these muffins and nut loaves just for the noon meal or for those young ones to snatch when they pass through my kitchen. I made some for Charles and for Jonas too."

"May I go with you when you deliver them?"

"Most certainly not."

The scarlet crept back into Sydney's face; then she saw Griselda laughing at her.

"I intend to take milk and buns to Abigail's room so she and the children can have a party this morning. And I want *you* to take a treat down to Jonas. Kersten will be along later this morning for a cooking lesson. Although—God forgive me for judging her—the girl has no real talent with cooking as far as I can see. I'll just send the sweet rolls back to the vicarage with her."

"Whenever I see her, Kersten is quite curious about the O'Reilly children. You'd think she was writing a report on them."

Mrs. Quigley slapped the flour from her hands. "Don't get yourself involved, Sydney. But you're right about Kersten. She's a pretty little thing with a dozen questions about Danny and Keeley when she works with me here in the kitchen. I just go about my business as though I never heard her."

As she spoke, she deftly arranged some bread and muffins on a china platter. She stepped back to admire her own work before laying a linen cloth on top. "Jonas will think you baked these for him. It worked with Arthur."

"I've never baked in my life."

"Too busy running that corporation of yours, huh? Don't get too busy and miss the lasting things of life. Jonas likes his sweets with cream and jam. I put a little on the platter. Now get a scurry on you and get down to his cottage before he's out mending the fence or ordering the gardeners around."

Sydney's hand flew to her hair, finger-combing it.

"You look just fine. Now go on. And tell him you want tea to go with the muffins. He can put a kettle over that fire-place of his, and it will be quite cozy for the two of you. And don't you come back until you've talked things out."

As Sydney passed in front of the manor, she saw Griselda standing in the window, smiling.

Sydney had never gone inside the cottage before. Now with her heart thumping and Mrs. Quigley's baked goods on a hand-painted china plate, she made her way over the flagstone path.

From the manor, she had a side view of the cottage, but approaching now, the whole place seemed concealed by over-hanging branches and high hedges. Coming around the taller hedges, she had her first real glimpse of the weaver's cottage. Two chimneys jutted above its low thatched roof, and ram-bling roses framed the door. More flowers lined the walkway to the stone steps, the sunlight making their lavender and pink petals glow. Off to her left came the sweet smell of honey-suckle and a more intoxicating odor of fermented apples.

A black umbrella sat in a brass urn on the side of the steps, within easy reach should an afternoon rain squall hit while she was visiting. She reached out to tap the brass knocker and realized that the door stood ajar.

"Jonas, it's Sydney."

Silence. Not even TopGun sniffed at the door.

As she tapped gently, the door swung back. "Anybody home?"

She stepped into the cluttered room cautiously. A dirty cup and saucer had been left on the lamp table, newspapers were strewn all over the floor, and Jonas's night slippers lay by the chair. Still the room, peculiarly masculine, had a cozy, lived-in satisfaction with an iron fireplace on the far wall, a hearth rug in front of it, and a glittering sword in its sheath hanging above the mantel.

From where she stood, she saw an answering machine that was blinking with a message of its own. She was lured across the room by the framed photograph of a pretty young woman on the mantel.

"Oh, hello!" The greeting came from behind her.

She whirled around to face Jonas and his black-and-white collie. Jonas's gaze strayed to the mantel and back to Sydney.

"The door was ajar. I just came in," she said matter-of-factly.

His thick black brows arched. "I see that you did."

She held out the plate. "I'm sorry for barging in on you, but I brought a peace offering. Griselda said you'd make us tea."

"I can't think of anything I'd like better than having tea with you." He grinned, shut the dog out, and tossed his jacket on the chair. "I'll stir the fire and put the kettle on."

"Griselda said you'd do it that way."

"What else did Griselda tell you?"

"She said to pretend I baked the muffins myself."

He laughed, a deep pleasant chuckle, a happy sound like those moments together on the hillside. He came to her side in a few long strides, and took the plate from her. As he peeked under the cloth, his eyes glowed. "Hum. As though I wouldn't recognize her baking. Smells great! And she remembered the jam and cream."

Setting the plate down, he bent to strike a match to the kindling. "This won't take long."

"Jonas, where did that sword above the mantel come from?"

The flames leaped around the kindling. He stood, his shoulder brushing hers. "That's the Admiral's ceremonial sword. It's the one he wore when he was in full dress uniform. When I was promoted to Lieutenant Commander, he gave it to me."

"You must be proud."

"I'm not likely to earn one myself. So, yes, I am proud to own it. And now with Dad ill—"

Her arm tingled at the twill of his sweater against it. "Don't underrate yourself." She looked up at him. "Abigail thinks you're as fine an officer as the Admiral."

Flecks of gray in his blue eyes overshadowed the sadness. "What else does Abigail say about me?"

Sydney laughed softly. "Over the last several weeks? That you're charming. Good looking. Intelligent. Trustworthy. That you'll go to the top. Even to a higher rank than your father."

"In other words, in Abby's eyes, I'm perfect?"

"Abigail tells me she has a thousand reasons for loving you."

He laughed. "Name just one."

"She's grateful to you for coming home."

"For the first time in my life, I think my dad needs me."

"He has always needed you. You just didn't know it."

"At first I thought about placing my father in a Navy residence. Now, I know I can't do it. I haven't worked out the details yet, but Dad has the right to live out his life here."

"I'm sure Lady Willoughby would want that."

He frowned. "And what do you know about Lady Willoughby?"

"Enough to know she would want you to take care of Abigail as well."

She moved away from him and inched her way along the wall, studying the pictures there. "If you keep the manor going for your father, does that mean you will have to give up the Navy?"

He followed her. "No. The Navy is my life. I'll make arrangements for others to come in and help Abigail and Griselda."

"And if Abby's heart gives out?"

"I would grieve for her, but there would be no regrets. With Dad I would grieve for an unhealed relationship. With Dad I never quite measured up, and now, with his health the way it is, we will never be able to set things right."

"When I'm with him, he talks about his son all the time."

"You seem to bring the best out of my father—and me. My father's plumb line was always ramrod straight, no bending, no allowance for error or deviation from the Willoughby standard. These days I no longer try to measure up."

"I don't believe that for a moment, Jonas. Coming home and sacrificing your chance to command a ship of your own is proof enough of that." She swallowed the rest of her curiosity and asked, "Were these all your ships?"

"Mine. Dad's. The other pictures were school photos taken at Gordonstoun and Dartmouth. And flying school."

She stopped by the picture from Gordonstoun. "You were really young there."

"I was head boy then. The lad on the playing field was our star rugby player. He won awards for rifle shooting." Jonas's face clouded. "I should have removed that picture, but he was one of Abigail's boys. He left a long time ago."

"Why?"

"I figured he left to fight with the IRA. It turned out that I was right."

She turned. "Is he Keeley's father? The missing Irishman?"

He said angrily, "Yes."

He reached up to remove the picture. Sydney put her hand on his arm. "Don't. Whatever politics came between the two of you, you were classmates and friends once. It's part of your past."

His voice was deep, his tone querulous. "You just don't understand the Irish question—the problem with the IRA."

"But I do understand the cry of a little girl. Someday you can show Keeley that picture. To Keeley he is not a terrorist. He's her father and she loves him. She's just a frightened, lonely five-year-old."

The kettle whistled persistently. He whirled to grab it. "I almost forgot. Get the muffins, would you? I'll pour the tea."

Moments later, Sydney gazed out the kitchen window with the teacup balanced in her hand. The magnificent English garden spread out from the house, past white marguerites that lay close to the ground. Far down the hill she could see an arbor of crimson roses. "The gardens are beautiful, Jonas."

"Abigail and my mother spent hours out there with the gardeners. Of course, Mother sometimes sat beneath one of the aspen or birch trees and watched Abigail work. But between them, they turned it into a place of beauty."

A place that she didn't want to leave behind. "Where were you when the work was being done?"

"Sitting on Mother's lap or spading the soil with Abigail."

"I'm going to hate leaving all of this."

"Then stay. Stay longer."

She laughed. "I have a corporation to run."

"I know. You keep reminding me."

Far to her left stood the stables and the grassland where the horses grazed. What had once been a moat in medieval times was a serene man-made lake now, a massive water tower beside it.

"The water tower mars this lovely setting," she observed.

"It's our reservoir for emergencies—a security factor in case of a dry season or fires. It's up to Lucas to keep the generator in mint condition. Boris is too old to tend it now."

Her eyes went back to the gardens. "Has it always been this lovely?"

"The gardens were overrun with weeds for a time during my long absence. And the manor was in a state of disrepair. I just wish Abby had told me she needed funds. But a year and a half ago someone left her money in a Swiss account, and she was able to get the manor repaired and the garden back the way she liked it."

The Broadshire account. Mother and Dad's gift to Abigail.

"Fortunately, I have Dad's power of attorney now. Abby won't lack for funds ever again. Everything you see and everything out front belongs to us. Two hundred and fifty acres of it."

He took her cup and set it aside. "All of this will belong to me someday, and I will have no one to share it with me if you go away. Sydney, I've been home for twelve hours trying to work up the courage to come and see you."

"Does it take courage?" she whispered.

"It takes courage to tell you what I want to tell you."

He was so close she could see the beat of his heart through his sweater. Could hear the thundering beat of her own.

"I don't want you to go away, Sydney. I love you."

He drew her closer and tilted her chin toward him. As he leaned down and his lips touched hers, the telephone rang.

A persistent ring like a trumpet blast, shattering their moment together.

Twenty-nine

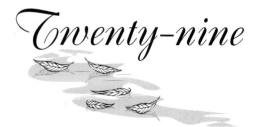

Captain McIntyre's voice roared over the wire. "Commander, there's a Learjet flying off course across Scotland with your friend Jock Hollinsworth in the pilot's seat."

Jonas snapped the television on. *For those just tuning in, we are following the flight of a runaway corporate jet. . . . Identity of the pilot is being withheld.*

"He's climbing erratically. That's not Jock's style."

"He's on automatic pilot. Air traffic requested escort when the jet veered off course. They've deployed two fighter jets."

"Are they from my old squadron?" Jonas asked.

"Yes, and they know Hollinsworth is on board. The wires into Northwood are jammed. The jets tracking him report no visible signs of life in the cabin and frosted windows in the cockpit."

"Then he's run out of oxygen. Is he flying alone?"

"He was scheduled to pick up two passengers in Stockholm. He was out of Helsinki on time but hasn't followed his flight pattern since leaving Stockholm. If the jet crosses over Ireland, they will shoot it down. Why the fool is logging hours on a commercial run, I'll never know."

The privately owned aircraft en route to London veered west over Newcastle . . . unconfirmed reports coming in believe the chase planes are waiting for the order to intercept and destroy.

On the screen, the twin-engine plane with its long wings looked like a white eagle soaring. Jock had called it a beauty—white with burgundy stripes and burgundy leather seats inside. It hadn't been ten days since Jonas had stood with Jock, talking about the future. Now he was waiting for his plane to run out of fuel and crash. Or, with one word from the Prime Minister, the jet pilots would hear the order to fire and blow the Learjet out of the sky.

The runaway jet is being tracked by fighter jets dispatched from a Scottish base. It is estimated that the plane drifting on automatic pilot will cross into Ireland within minutes. . . . The name of the Navy pilot is still being withheld.

"Captain, Jock's wife may be pregnant. She's in London."

"She's here at Northwood . . . waiting out the end with us."

When the call ended, Jonas looked at Sydney. "Jock is on board. They lost contact with him shortly after takeoff."

Sydney's face turned ghostly. In three strides he was at her side, his arm around her. "Sydney, nothing can be done. But Jock is not in pain. I promise you that. Within seconds, he'd be unconscious from oxygen starvation. A window blowout. A broken seal. Something caused decompression. Without oxygen, he would be euphoric one moment, disoriented and unconscious the next."

As he stood by her side, Jonas noticed the light blinking on the answering machine. He pushed the play button and heard "Friday, 9:25 A.M.," and then Jock's voice, "Commander, it's Jock. I have to talk to you. Where are you?"

Jock went on muttering. "I leave Stockholm at 9:10, en route to London. No . . . I think the plane took off with unwanted cargo. If I don't make it—" He started humming.

"Jonas, why would he spend half of a phone message humming a song? He knows your anger with the IRA. He's too close a friend to aggravate you with an Irish lyric," Sydney said.

"Jock did crazy things."

"But Kathleen is the one who would want to know when he was taking off—so she could meet him when he arrived in London. What did he mean unwanted cargo? Your friend wasn't transporting drugs, was he?"

Nettled, Jonas said, "Of course not. He did things like that—whistling, passing along jokes between us with a song. On some of our routine flights, Jock would hum some message. Something that just the two of us understood."

"But this time he sounded desperate. It sounds like the plane he was supposed to be flying took off without him. Jonas, he sang that same song at the picnic."

She tried to recall the lyrics as Jock had sung them and could only grab at a phrase or two. Something about green leaves in December and fragrant roses dying. And snows covering a land that had never known freedom. She remembered Jock telling them that the Irish thrived on laughter and music, yet their land did not know freedom, and only the fast-flowing rivers of their land ran free. She poked the replay button on Jonas's answering machine and listened to Jock again. In the middle of a sentence the message ended abruptly as though someone had cut him off.

His voice cracked as he asked, "What difference does it make if he was humming an Irish lyric?" Jonas asked. "Any moment, he'll never sing again. Whatever happened on board, he didn't have time to don an oxygen mask. That Learjet is on automatic."

"For how long?" she whispered.

"Until it crashes. But they'll shoot it down rather than risk a crash landing in a populated city in Ireland. One word from the Prime Minister and they will blow Jock out of the sky."

The runaway plane is over the Irish Sea, nearing the coast of the Emerald Isle.

"No, Jock. No." Jonas groaned as the jet lost its cruising altitude and plunged in a spiraling arc through the clouds toward earth, leaving a vapor trail behind her. It plunged into the sea, the twisted debris surfacing moments after the plane dove into its watery grave. The chase fighters lowered, circling above the sea, and then as thousands of listeners watched, they changed course and headed back toward Scotland.

Jonas didn't move. Sydney switched off the television and hit the replay button on the answering machine again. "Friday, 9:25 A.M.," the mechanical voice said. And then Jock's voice, "Commander, it's Jock. I have to talk to you. Where are you? . . . Jonas, pick up that phone . . . I don't have long. . . . We're still holed up in Stockholm. I may have lost the dart game. . . . Scheduled to pick up two passengers in Stockholm, but the men who showed up—" The message ended abruptly.

"Jonas, what time did Jock's plane take off for London?"

"Nine-ten. And on schedule."

For the third time she hit the replay button and the mechanical voice with the nasal twang came through clearly. "Friday, 9:25 A.M. . . ."

He stared at her. "Jock called after the plane took off. If he wasn't on board, then someone commandeered that jet," he said.

"So what happened?"

"Everything was normal out of Helsinki. Whatever happened took place in Sweden where he was supposed to pick up two passengers."

"Was he telling you the destination—to a land that didn't have freedom—where only the rivers ran free?"

He fixed his gaze on the BBC telecast, still repeating the same news. "Only a fool would try passing deliberately into Irish air space—and refuse to respond to traffic control. He'd try bluffing first. Declare an emergency. No, whoever was in that cabin was unconscious. Jock may have been telling us that the theft was accomplished by Irish terrorists. A plane like that would be an asset to the IRA. You're brilliant, sweetheart."

He whirled around, grabbed his phone, and called McIntyre. "Captain," he said, when McIntyre answered. "I don't think Jock Hollinsworth was on board that jet."

"Don't be a fool, Willoughby."

"He left a message on my answering machine fifteen minutes after the Learjet took off. Someone else was flying that plane."

"You sound certain."

"A gut reaction. There may be an Irish tie-in. When Jock and his wife visited us here in Stow-on-the-Woodland, we had dinner at Chutman's Pub. Jock challenged just about everyone to a game of darts—and he talked freely about his trip. Someone at the pub may have wanted that plane more than he did."

Sydney strained to hear the captain's answer. "You're crazy, Willoughby."

"Sir, the plane took off from Stockholm out of a private airstrip. We need to start looking there. Captain, may I have your permission to fly up there where Jock was last seen?"

"Is that wise, Willoughby?"

"He was my wingman—my best friend. Jock would do the same for me."

"All right. I've spoken to the chief inspector in the area. I told him I would send one of my own men to undertake an investigation. But if something goes wrong, we will deny sending you there. But, Willoughby, if you find him, accompany his body back to the base in Scotland."

"For proper burial?" he asked.

"No, for an autopsy."

"I don't intend to bring Jock back in a body bag. I expect to find him alive."

"There are reports that his uncle is under suspicion."

"Rodney Christopher wouldn't harm his nephew."

"Greed can be a strange bedfellow. Rumors have it that Christopher has Irish ties. For all we know, Jock Hollinsworth may have been scheduled to transport arms to the IRA."

Discovering Jock's body came within hours, more speedily than anyone expected. With the quick arrest and confession of Rodney Christopher, Jonas and the inspection team were led to an old warehouse close to the private airstrip in Stockholm where Jock was last seen. Jonas dropped down beside his friend's bruised and battered body. Jock lay in an embryo curl, blood crusted at his mouth. But he was alive.

Jonas gripped his hand. "Jock, you're going to be okay."

"My wife?"

"We'll get word to Kathleen right away. Sydney is with her."

"Did my uncle make it?"

"He wasn't flying the plane, Jock. Someone else was."

"Impossible. He'd never let anyone touch that plane." His voice faded. "I have to talk to him."

"No can do. They just arrested your uncle."

Jock tried to open his eyes. "For what?"

"For attempting to transport illegal arms into Ireland. And for conspiracy to transport his Learjet into the hands of the IRA—at the risk of your life."

"No, Jonas—he wouldn't do that."

"I'm sorry, old man. But we've always been up front with each other. Your uncle has already confessed."

He tried to lift his head and failed miserably. "Why?" he groaned.

"He was secretly involved in the Irish movement. But when I told him you were missing, he broke down. If he hadn't told us about the warehouse, we might not have reached you in time."

Jonas beckoned to the medical team. The medics tried to roll Jock to a more comfortable position. "Don't. Don't move me. I—I have to talk to Jonas . . . I told Uncle Rodney that something was wrong. The next thing I remember was a blow to my head."

Jock's body jerked as he was given an injection. He struggled to speak. "I think the plane was in the air when I called you. . . . All I could do was leave a message on your machine. And then . . . two friends of my uncle broke in on me. The last thing I remember is being tossed in the back of the truck." His speech slurred. "You'll call Kathleen—"

"Right away."

As they lifted Hollinsworth on the stretcher, the Swedish inspector said, "He looks bad. Do you think your friend will make it?"

Jonas flashed a grim smile. "He'll make it. He has a score to settle with his uncle. And his reputation to salvage for working with that man."

"Can I give you a lift somewhere, Commander?"

"To the hospital. As soon as I know Jock is going to be all right, I'll head back to England. To his wife—and my girl."

In the days that followed, Jonas slipped into a brooding silence. As they walked together among the primrose bushes, Sydney said, "Now that I know that Jock will recover, I've made my reservation. I'm leaving Thursday, Jonas."

He whirled around to face her and gripped her arms. "Is there nothing I can do to make you stay?"

"Nothing. I think it's best for both of us. So much has happened—you need time to sort it all out. Abigail. Your dad. Jock."

"And you. You're the one who matters to me now."

"We'll stay in touch. We'll write—"

As they resumed walking, she linked her arm in his and pressed her head against his shoulder. "We knew I would go home someday."

"But I want you to stay." He leaned down and kissed her on the top of her head. "I love you. It won't be the same here without you."

"You won't be here, Jonas. You're going back to North-wood next week. Things will settle down to normal. And Dr. Wallis and Charles promised Abigail that they would arrange for more staff to help Griselda."

His fingers tightened around hers. "I'm grateful, Sydney."

As they reached the manor, Charles plodded up the stone steps. "Charles!" she called. "What are you doing here?"

He turned, his face old and tired, his blue eyes pale and heavy lidded. "I have come with bad news for Abigail."

"No, Charles," Jonas warned. "That Learjet crash and Jock's injuries have upset her enough."

Sydney nudged Jonas. "Charles, Jock is better, but you look as though you haven't slept for days."

"I haven't." He hesitated. "Jeff and Chandler insisted that I come now. It's about Conon O'Reilly."

Sydney's grip silenced Jonas. "What about Conon?" she asked.

"He's dead."

"Dead!"

"He nodded. "You were right, Sydney, when you said he was staying in the vicarage with me." He peered over the tops of his glasses at Jonas. "I kept him in the Jacobean room. Abigail told me that you and the other boys played there when you were young, Jonas. Before my time at St. Michael's."

Jonas's gaze turned icy. "I trusted you, Charles. But you protected an Irish terrorist. You and Abigail?"

"She knows nothing. The last she saw of Conon was the night she had her heart attack. May I see Abigail alone, please?"

"Let him, Jonas. We'll be with you shortly."

Twenty minutes later, when Sydney and Jonas stepped into Abigail's room, Charles was putting the communion cups aside. Abigail held out a hand to each of them. "How is Jock?"

Jonas squeezed her fingers. "Better. Kathleen is with him."

"Charles took communion with me." She smiled, a serene look on her face. Turning to him, she said, "I'm ready to hear the bad news now that the children are with me. It's about Conon, isn't it?"

Charles nodded. "He's gone, Abigail. He was seriously injured, but he refused to see a doctor. He died from those wounds."

311

"Was he with you all that time?"

"I wasn't there the night he died. Friends buried him when I was in London with the archbishop."

"Then he was buried without a funeral."

Jonas turned livid. "He didn't deserve a funeral, Abigail."

Lucas Sullivan sat at his shortwave radio and twisted the dials. The crash of the Learjet just short of the Irish coastline had been a personal loss. What had gone wrong? What did he know of decompression and hypoxia? And what had become of Rodney Christopher? Had he been arrested? No matter where Lucas tuned in, the plane crash was stale news. Yesterday, Jock Hollinsworth's face had been sprawled across the television screen and his condition upgraded from critical to satisfactory. The investigation of the crash site was ongoing. How long would it take them to realize that weapons destined for the IRA were part of the debris?

Fools, he thought. *Better if it had been Hollinsworth dead, not two of my good men.*

Joseph Hollinsworth had outwitted him. Would he link the plane to Lucas? Not likely, but he might trace talks of his plane back to the picnic at Stow-on-the-Woodland or the dart game at Chutman's Pub. Then Jonas Willoughby and Jock Hollinsworth would begin to put it all together. It seemed like everything began falling apart the day he found Sydney Barrington's riding stick in his room. What had she told Jonas? He had mistrusted her from the day she walked into the manor. He despised her now. But why had she chosen to keep silent about his shortwave radio set?

For his own safety he must move on. But first he would send one last message to Belfast. And then he would destroy the stables. He could not risk moving the technical equipment in time, and he regretted that his actions might cost the life of the Admiral. He had, after all, a fondness for the old man.

Conon was another burden. Convincing Charles that Conon was dead and buried was the best way to ward off any questions from Charles and the Church of England. He didn't care what they did with the dotty clergyman. They'd already put him out to pasture when they sent him to the smallest of flocks here in Stow-on-the-Woodland. What else could they do but retire him?

Lucas's plans for Stow-on-the-Woodland had failed, but his men were strong enough to start over somewhere else. Their cause was greater than any peace negotiations. He found satisfaction that the destruction of the stables would forever cut off the tunnel entry into the bottom floor of the manor. But he could not bring himself to destroy the splendid horses.

He had rescued the ammunition from the stockpiles hidden in the tunnel. The thought that the heat of fire would cause the tunnel entry to cave in gave him pleasure. He gathered up the discs from the computer and placed his gun collection in the back of the lorry. He would order the schoolmaster to drive the truck to the north country. As the manor was slowly enshrouded in darkness, Lucas led the horses from the stable and tethered them one by one on a high hill.

He turned to the young sheepherder who met him there. "Don't take Commander Willoughby's stallion."

"But he's a thoroughbred, Lucas."

"The stallion is as British as Jonas. Leave him." He rubbed the neck of the chestnut stallion, his favorite, and saddled him. "Take this one to the hills until I am ready to leave. O'Reilly may not live long enough to ride out with me, but take a second horse just in case."

"And the pony?"

"The pony belongs to Keeley O'Reilly."

At midnight he spread stacks of hay through the stables and around the circumference of his room. In the last half hour he sorted through his papers, stowed the most important ones in his briefcase, and left the others to burn. He saturated his mattress with gasoline and leaned it against the computer and wireless systems. He set fire to the wastebasket, knowing that it would smolder, giving him time to escape. Then, emptying the can of gasoline on the stairwell, he descended for the last time. Coils of smoke trailed from his room. He was going out in style. He struck another match to one of the stalls and fled.

Plumes of smoke darkened over Stow-on-the-Woodland as Lucas made his way stealthily to the primary school where Conon was growing more restless than ever. He considered leaving him behind, letting him really die, but he could not do that to Keeley. The child's father was dying, but it was better for both of them to return to Ireland. He owed Conon O'Reilly that much.

Thirty

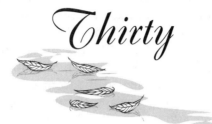

Barrington Enterprises won the primary bid on the aircraft carriers, but the win did little to lift Sydney's sinking spirit. She stared down at the half-packed suitcases. Once she left the Cotswolds, she might never see Jonas again, not until the carriers slipped into the water at the Jarrow Shipyard in Tyne. He promised to be there for the launching, but going on without him now left her wobbly-kneed. Never had she loved anyone as she loved Jonas Willoughby. From that first day by the primroses, he had snipped at her heart strings with those pruning shears.

She flattened another blouse in the suitcase as someone banged repeatedly on her door. "Fire! Fire, Miss Barrington!"

She flung the door back. Boris's face flushed with excitement. "We have to get Miss Abigail to safety! The stables are burning; come, quickly!"

He shuffled off as close to a run as she had seen him do. She shoved her bare feet into her shoes and followed him.

"Where's Jonas? Where's Lucas?" she cried. "Is Lucas—"

"No one has seen Lucas, and Jonas went for his father."

"Boris, where are the fire trucks?"

He stared at her, dumbfounded. "We have no fire trucks. Just the water tower, if we can get it to work."

They found Abigail standing by her bed, trembling. Boris grabbed a coat from her closet and forced her arms in it.

"The children, Boris?"

"Griselda and Santos went for the children, Miss Abigail."

"Sit down," Sydney said gently. "Let me get your shoes on."

"No, get my riding boots from the closet. They should still fit me. Boris, grab blankets and wet washcloths for the children. They'll have trouble breathing."

"No," Sydney cautioned. "We have to get you outside."

They practically lifted her and ran. Abigail's booted toes dragged across the parquet to the front door. Plumes of smoke rose above the village as they rushed down the stone steps.

"I forgot my medicine," she coughed. "The Admiral! Sydney, Boris go for the Admiral. I'll be all right."

"Jonas went for his father," Boris assured her.

As they rounded the side of the house, they heard the crackling roar of the fire and saw the stables engulfed in flames. They found Griselda and the children in the primrose garden and gently lowered Abigail on a wooden bench.

Griselda stood in her flannel nightgown, an arm around two of the children. She stared transfixed at the shooting flames, unaware that the air had thickened with the smell of smoke. The schoolmaster and several stronger men had converged on the water tower, attaching hoses to the valves. As the water hit the fire, it sizzled into steam. Others beat the flames with towels and blankets, trying to halt the rapid spread of fire through the tall grass as the wind swept the burning embers toward the manor.

Keeley flew to Sydney. "My pony, Sydney. My pony."

Gregor's dark eyes were like neon lights in the flames. "Your pony's safe. The schoolmaster told me. He said someone turned the horses out of their stalls before the fire started."

Sydney was shocked. If someone had set the horses free, the fire was no accident. "Is Lucas fighting the fire?" she asked.

Gregor shrugged. "No one has seen him."

She put her free arm around him and thought of the terror he had known in Kosovo. "Are you all right, Gregor?"

He leaned against her, his dark eyes brimming with tears. "Griselda told me to be brave for the little children."

She ruffled his hair. "Gregor, have you seen Jonas yet?"

"Him and TopGun went back for the Admiral." He turned his head and cried out with delight, "There's Jonas!"

Jonas struggled toward them with his father's limp body in his arms and the dog close on his heels. He was breathing heavily as he reached them. Glaring at Abigail, he asked, "Did you have to go so far to protect Conon?"

"Don't even think that, Jonas." She made a place for the Admiral on the bench beside her, and Jonas eased his father down. Then he ran to join the other men.

Smoke drove the firefighters back. With a deafening rumble the roof and one wall of the stables caved in. The roar of the fire and crackling sound of walls collapsing terrified Sydney. Above the popping explosions inside the stable, she heard the grinding gasp of the power generator nearby. The sound faded. Someone cursed. Boris tried to fire the generator again. It sputtered to action and in minutes the water pump flowed freely.

The men from the village shouted as the flames leaped toward the manor. "Get the children farther back!"

"Griselda," Sydney urged, "we must get the children back!"

Jonas shrugged in disgust as he ran past them. "She doesn't hear you, Sydney. Even if she did, she wouldn't move away. This is her home. She'd have nowhere else to go."

"Griselda!" Sydney cried again. "Let's move farther back."

She was too dazed, paralyzed. Abigail went to her and gently said, "Griselda, it's Abigail."

"It's like the London blitz, Abby. Are the planes coming?"

"There are no planes, no bombs. The stables are on fire. We have to keep the children safe."

Danny's scream brought her to her senses. She gathered him to her and moved back as more plumes of smoke rose above them.

"I forgot my medicine," Abigail said, her voice raspy. "And the blankets for the children. The smoke is making it hard for me to breathe. We need wet cloths to put over our faces."

317

Moments later Sydney asked, "Where's Gregor?"

"Oh, no. He must have gone for my medicine."

"I'll find him." The smoke burned Sydney's eyes as she ran back toward the house, slipping and sliding where the water had turned the ground to mud. She was near the west wing now and saw tiny flames crawling up the side of the building toward the Admiral's room. She heard the sound of shattered glass as the windows blew. The flames licked higher, catching the eaves on fire.

"Jonas!" she screamed. "The house is on fire!"

They were dragging a hose toward the west wing as she stumbled up the front steps and found Gregor on the top one, crying. He clutched Abigail's medicine bottle in one hand, a fist full of wet cloths in the other. He thrust the cloths at her. "I'm afraid, Sydney."

"We all are. It took a brave boy to go for her medicine."

She took only a second to hug him against her, and then they were running through the smoke-filled night back to the others. As they reached them, the rest of the stable walls tumbled in and only the blackened silhouette of the old stables remained.

As the smoke rose, ash fell back on them. "The worst is over," Jonas said. "It'll take another two or three hours for the fire to die out. I've left the schoolmaster in charge."

Jonas looked exhausted, his face covered with soot. One sweater sleeve was torn away, the hairs on one arm singed. He squeezed Sydney's shoulder. "I'm glad you're all right. Thank God my forefathers were wise enough to set up a water system."

Abigail's hand still rested comfortably on the Admiral's arm, but his groggy indifference troubled Jonas. The old man's eyelids hung heavy, and his speech had slurred.

"Lucas?" the Admiral asked. "Is he safe? We have a ship to fire up. We're going on winter patrol off the coast of Ireland."

"Lucas is gone, Dad."

The vacant eyes stared at him in the darkness. "Did Lucas do this after all I've done for him?"

"Dad, why would you say that?"

He frowned, searching for his answer. "He stole money from my black box the other night. He thought I was sleeping."

Abigail patted the Admiral's hand. "Tobias, I'm still here to take care of you."

Jonas shook his head. "Don't worry, Abby. Dad's confused."

Sydney said, "Lucas is the only man in the whole village who missed the flames shooting in the air. Where was he? I think your father's right. Lucas had constant access to the stables. Who else would have saved Keeley's pony and your stallion?"

Jonas glanced where the stables once stood. "You don't think—"

"No; we would have heard him screaming. But you don't scream when you're setting a fire."

His anger roiled. "You're reading it wrong, Sydney. Lucas served with the Royal Navy. He's been Dad's steward for twenty years. He wouldn't do a thing like this."

Exasperated, she said, "Tomorrow ask your commanding officer and his intelligence team to sift through the ashes. You'll find evidence of a sophisticated computer system and a sender and receiver radio set. Why would the Admiral's caregiver need those? I know he had them. I was in his room once." When his eyes hardened, she said hastily, "I was with Keeley."

"He disliked children."

"But he felt a particular bond with Keeley—and you know he loved horses. I think he let all the horses go free before he started the fire. You can stop blaming everything on Abigail. Abigail didn't burn the stables. She doesn't even have the strength to walk that far."

As they stared at the charred ruins, Sydney said, "I'm sorry, Jonas. It's just that Abigail loves you too much to ever hurt you. And you seem blind to her love."

He struggled to bring his eyes level with Sydney's. "We may never know how the fire started. Now help me. We must get my father back inside."

"Take the Admiral to my room," Abigail told him. "Tobias can sleep there, and I will sit with him. Griselda—"

The housekeeper stood shivering in her nightgown, a shawl thrown around her shoulders—the children huddled beside her.

"Griselda."

She turned and faced her old friend. "I'm here, Abigail."

"Would you take the children inside while Boris and Jonas assess the damage. And, Sydney, make some tea for all of us."

"That's my job, Abby," Griselda protested. "I made some sweet bread and cookies. Really, I should make the tea."

"Not tonight. Tonight I want you to be with the children. I want you to rest. Sydney will check in on you later."

An hour later Jonas discarded his ash-covered boots at the front door. The boots were water-logged, the soles black from soot. He went directly to Abigail's room and found her spooning hot tea between the Admiral's lips.

Sir James swallowed, but his gaze remained vacant. There wasn't a flicker when Jonas entered. "Is Dad still dazed?"

"Lucas may have given him some sleeping medication—enough to keep him quiet when Lucas left the room."

Jonas's jaw jerked. "Griselda keeps his medicine in the kitchen."

Abigail smiled at him, her eyes sad. "Lucas knew his way around the kitchen. Now, we'll say no more of it."

His gaze traversed the room, searching for Sydney. She came from the bathroom, a cup of scalding tea in her hands. She kissed his sooty cheek and handed him the tea. "Tell us what you've found, Jonas."

For a second he couldn't take his eyes from her. She was leaving soon, and he had done nothing to stop her from going away. He swallowed his pride, his yearning. "The stables are gone but still smoldering—and two of the stallions unaccounted for."

"Lost in the fire?" Sydney asked.

"We don't know. Some of the men offered to stay through the night. They'll hose down anything that sparks again."

Her eyes still locked with his. "There's a wide patch of destruction between the house and stables. The walls of the kitchen were seared and some windows blown out from the heat."

He glanced back at his father asleep against Abigail's thick pillows. "The west wing suffered considerable water damage. Some of Dad's Navy pictures are destroyed, and the rug is ruined. I'm glad he's resting. It would break his heart to see how close Lady Willoughby's property came to being destroyed."

Someone cleared his throat behind Jonas. He turned and saw Charles filling the doorway, a prayer book in his hands.

"How dare you come here. Wasn't the message you brought to us last night enough? Do you think I appreciated your telling us that Conon O'Reilly was gone?"

"I've come as your friend, Jonas."

"The friend of Her Majesty? The friend of Stow-on-the-Woodland? You hid a terrorist. Have you no conscience?"

"My conscience battled me all the while. But no matter what you think of me, I saw Conon O'Reilly as a prodigal in need of a Father."

Jonas's bitterness spewed out. "So you wanted to be his father? His own father failed him pitifully."

"I wanted God to be his Father."

"Charles," Abigail said, "You are welcome as long as I am here. But knowing you, Reverend, you always come with a purpose in mind. Perhaps even with a prayer."

"Abigail, I was thinking how fortunate we all are—"

"Fortunate?" Jonas exploded. "We just had a fire."

The catch in Charles's voice stilled him. "Dr. Wallis set up an emergency clinic on the south wing. Two of our villagers were overcome with smoke inhalation. One of the sheep farmers singed the hair on his face and arms. The pub owner has burns on both hands. They'll blister, but he'll be fine in a few weeks."

"So you expect me to be grateful?" Jonas asked.

"Jonas, the whole village turned out to help you, and my American houseguests were out there working hard beside the other men with no thought to their own safety."

"And Santos?" Abigail asked. "Where was he?"

"There as well, with smoke smudges on his cheeks and his clothes reeking of smoke. I saw a new Santos this evening, Abigail. A selfless man working hard to prevent the flames reaching the art work at Broadshire Manor."

"Poor Santos. I never even thought of the art treasures."

"Just about your children," Charles said kindly. "They were always first in your mind, Abigail. You left an imprint on Santos's life as well. That's why he's here—why he stayed with the firefighters this evening instead of tearing down the tapestries from the walls or carrying paintings to safety."

Charles's shoulders bent forward. "I've been with Griselda and the children. They're frightened, but she's with them. It was Griselda who said we all have need of healing in this house."

Jonas glared back. "No one from the manor was hurt."

"Since the night of Abigail's heart attack you have all been hurting. It's time to forgive one another. For past hurts." For a moment his eyes settled on Abigail and the Admiral. "To undo the past. To right the wrongs. The villagers—most of us—think Lucas was involved. I think the fire was more than a warning. More than the destructive act of one devious man. And until we know for certain—"

Jonas would have none of it. "All the sermons in the world can't erase the fact that you hid an IRA terrorist. What was wrong with you—the IRA killed your daughter."

"But I know Louise would not turn a wounded man out on the streets. I can understand if you cannot forgive me,

Jonas, but I've come to ask you to hold a proper burial for Conon."

"Why didn't you give him a proper ceremony, as you call it?"

"I told you. I was in London with the archbishop, giving an accounting of harboring a wounded man in the vicarage."

"Were you completely honest with the archbishop, Charles?"

"I asked for time to consider the matter. And because of my long time with the church, he granted it. When I came back to the village, Lucas told me Conon was dead and buried."

"Lucas knew he was there?"

"Yes." Charles rubbed his hands distractedly. "Conon had a glimmering of faith in the end. He was born a Catholic. He'd forgotten all of that, but he still remembered Abigail praying for him. Louise was killed on his father-in-law's farm. That was shock enough, but when he learned that Louise was your fiancée, he was devastated. Even in illness, he wanted your friendship."

"I don't need your sermons, Charles."

"No, you need a Father's healing. A Father's restoration."

"My father never qualified."

"Because you wouldn't let him," Abigail defended.

"This morning as I walked about the village—knowing that my church will be taken from me—I climbed to the highest knoll and looked down on St. Michael's and knew that if I must, I will give it up. What I did for Conon came from my heart."

Abigail cried in alarm. "We won't let the archbishop send you away and close up St. Michael's again. If the archbishop fails us, no wonder Conon couldn't believe that a God of mercy was waiting to forgive him."

Jonas opened his mouth, but a look from Abigail silenced him. "Can't you understand, Jonas, both good and pain slip through God's fingers. You wanted to avenge Louise's death, but has it made you happy?"

"Where was God when Louise died?"

Charles said, "I must believe that a merciful God was in Ireland that day with my daughter—waiting for the angels themselves to carry her Home. The prophet Hosea says that God wants acknowledgment of Himself, Jonas. How long will you go on ignoring favor with a forgiving God?"

Jonas's eyes sought Sydney's again. She came to him and brushed back the ruffled strands of hair that the wind and fire had unsettled. "I think what Jonas really wants to know is whether your church will allow you to conduct a service for an enemy of this country?"

"Whatever objections they may have, it seems to me that every prodigal needs a listening ear—a gentle farewell."

Abigail's hand was motionless now. "Charles, if I had known that Conon was with you, you know I would have gone to him."

"I would have had to carry you there," he teased. "The Jacobean room is dark and airless. You would have wanted him removed from there at once."

"You did your best."

"The archbishop doesn't agree. I talked with him by phone once I knew that Conon was gone and admitted that I had broken the laws of the church protecting him. The church intends to retire me to the North country. So what we do for Conon must be done quickly, Abigail."

In a flash of anger, she said, "I'll deal with the archbishop later. For now, Keeley and Danny O'Reilly are my concern."

Jonas steeled himself. Her words were directed to him now. "Conon was one of my boys. When I took his children in, I should have protected their father as well. But I didn't want to hurt you, Jonas. I haven't even found the courage to tell them that he's gone forever."

"I'll tell them," he offered huskily.

"No, I won't burden you with the children, Jonas."

Charles wrung his hands. "No matter what Jonas decides, Abigail, you and I will meet at Conon's grave—say two days from now and we'll have a memorial for a lost boy."

"I'll stay over long enough for the funeral," Sydney said. "And I think Jeff and Chandler will come."

"I'd have Kersten make us a funeral tea, Abigail, but I'm about to lose my house help. Last night she told me she is flying back to the States with Jeffrey."

The lamplight formed shadows on Abigail's frown. "Then something's going right. What will you do, Jonas?"

"I can't honor an enemy with a public funeral."

"Not honor, Jonas," Charles challenged. "Bury properly. Perhaps your conscience would let you do that. Have you called your commanding officer about Lucas yet? I can give them all the confirmation they need. Lucas was angry about the Northern Ireland agreements. Furious with his comrades for laying down arms."

His expression held a measure of hope. "The cry for peace is much stronger than Lucas expected. But he's a strong leader. If he can get a small faction to follow him, one bombing would destroy everything."

Abigail pointed to a phone near her. "The lines are still open to Northwood. The fire didn't destroy the connection."

Jonas crossed the room with Sydney at his side. He wiped his palms on his trousers and took the phone. As he dialed in the number, she kissed him on the cheek. "Things will work out, Jonas. You can build the stables again."

"Better that I turn over the property to the National Trust and let them restore Broadshire Manor to its previous glory."

"We'll see. One step at a time."

"Will you stay with me, Sydney?" he asked.

"Until Conon's funeral."

"And after that?"

He was so close that the tweed of his torn sweater brushed her arm. His own smell of smoke and burning overpowered her usual French scent. She looked exhausted with rivulets

325

of tears making uneven streams down her sooty face. Yearning for her gripped him.

"Yes—yes. Captain McIntyre? Commander Willoughby here."

He gave a brisk description of all that had happened. The fire. The possible betrayal of his father's steward. Conon's death.

"Is your father—and everyone else safe?"

"Captain, the Admiral is resting. Some of the firefighters were hurt, but no one at the manor was injured, although Lucas Sullivan must have intended harm to all of us."

"He was a classic sleeper, Commander. Living right there and using the manor as his headquarters."

"He always talked against the IRA dissidents."

"It's a small faction like Lucas who could ruin everything that has taken place at the conference table. Neither side wants any more violence in Northern Ireland. We don't want anything that will threaten the Ulster peace. That's why we wanted to find O'Reilly and that group still holding out with him."

And then Jonas—a proud, arrogant man as Charles had called him—said, "Sir, I'll resign my commission if it seems advisable. We had our man, Captain. A man I trusted and confided in, and I was too blind to see him. . . . He's gone, sir."

McIntyre's answer boomed back over the line. "We're not taking any resignations this year. Don't worry. Lucas Sullivan won't go far, Commander. We've been checking his background ever since my visit with the Admiral."

"You questioned his loyalty then?"

"Your father was alert enough to warn us. He told me when he was first retired a lot of gold braid came for visits. When the visitors dwindled, Mr. Sullivan didn't like it."

"But, sir, Sullivan was with the Royal Navy for years."

"He used the Service and your father to gain what he wanted. Stow-on-the-Woodland was a nice, quiet place for him to plan his war against any peace agreement. We believe now that Sullivan counted on the top brass from the Royal Navy dropping by for unexpected visits. He may have counted on being in on bits of information passed along whenever any of us visited the Admiral. Cordon off the area, Commander. We'll have military advisors there by morning. I want them to go through Sullivan's quarters."

"Sir, the stables were completely destroyed. Everything's in ashes. I should have known. You said it would be someone close at hand. Forgive me, sir, for not realizing that Lucas was using the Admiral and Broadshire Manor as headquarters."

He had used the words, and knew he was on the verge of seeking deeper forgiveness. He wanted inner peace. Tomorrow—or the next day—before Sydney flew home perhaps they could go to the vicarage together and talk with Charles. In spite of the heavy weight he was carrying this evening, Charles Rainford-Simms was a man of peace and joy. The peace and joy that Jonas needed. Something that he wanted for Sydney as well.

Captain McIntyre's blustery voice drew him back. "They'll sift through those ashes, Jonas. We have Sullivan's Navy records. His thumbprints. His photo. His history. We'll find him. And if he has sympathetic contacts there in the village, we'll find them. We're good at the waiting game. I just hope you're back to flying that Sea Harrier of yours or commanding your own ship by then. Good night, Commander."

Thirty-one

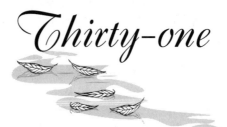

Sydney dressed in a striking dark suit for the walk down to St. Michael's churchyard. Somehow, she could not bring herself to think of Conon O'Reilly as dead, not even with that memory of a gaunt young man on the hillside with an Irish twang and a catch in his voice when he spoke of his children. As sick as he was, she had thought him crafty enough to make his way safely out of Stow-on-the-Woodland. Was she the only one who questioned his sudden death and burial?

As she wandered down the wide hall, her high heels tapping against the parquet flooring, Jonas said, "Sydney."

She turned and met his smile. "Hi, you're not dressed for the memorial service yet."

"Come sit with me outside by the fountain."

She went gladly, happy that the white bench was too small for three people. "I've dreaded this day, Jonas. Mostly for the children and because Abigail is hurting."

"She's a strong woman."

"You say that when her heart is as weak as it is?"

"I'm talking about Abigail's inner strength. There's no flutter or missed beats to that one. No mother wants to bury her child, and Conon was as much one of hers as the rest of us."

You more than any of them.

"I have something to tell you," he said. "I won't be taking Edmund Gallagher to court. There's no need for that now."

"What happened?"

"I called his law offices in London this morning and spoke to the senior partners. Edmund Gallagher shot himself yesterday."

She felt a sudden chill. "Gallagher is dead?"

"Blackstone and Rentley threatened to have him disbarred. His career was over. What probably disgraced him even more was the loss of face here with old friends."

"Abigail would not push to that extreme."

"No, there were others who lost great sums through Edmund's conniving. He tended to pick on widows with no immediate families. Thanks to your friend Jeff, Blackstone and Rentley were warned in time to correct these errors. They've combed through Edmund's files for days now. Once they told Edmund his career was over, he went back into his office and took his father's revolver out of the safe. For Edmund, greed was his downfall."

"Does Abigail know?"

"I just came from telling her. That on top of the memorial for Conon—and she's in for a rough day. But she's determined to walk down to the church on her own feet."

"We'll have to carry her back."

"Griselda is with her. They're old friends. But I don't know whether Keeley and Danny understand what's happening."

"Abigail and I talked with them last evening. Keeley cried so I took her to my room and Danny stayed with Abigail."

"No wonder you both look exhausted, Sydney."

"Little children don't stay on their side of the bed."

"This morning Abby said she had already lost a son, and losing Conon was more than she could bear. I'm not certain what she meant since he is the first of her hidden children to die."

She touched the back of his hand and ran her fingers gently over it. "Someday you'll understand."

She glanced at his khaki shorts and cambric cloth shirt. "Are you going to the church, Jonas? You can walk down with me."

"You go along. I have something else to do."

"Your father is all right alone. He's so much better now."

"Boris has him up in the chair by the window so he can watch what's going on. He thinks it's a funeral at sea. He's commanding everything from his bridge. Last night when we talked he finally remembered who Conon O'Reilly was. It's hard having Dad slip in and out of the present, but he had tears in his eyes when he told me, 'That boy and I used to walk by the Windrush.'"

"Did they?"

"Yes. A long time ago. Conon idolized my dad. I'm not sure why he and Dad hit it off so well, but they did. Abigail says Conon always wanted to be a Willoughby."

"You can't forgive Conon, can you, Jonas?"

He looked away, but she wasn't certain he was seeing anything beyond the fountain. Whatever had touched him—whatever he was struggling with inside—he would have to face his adversaries alone while the rest of them were gone.

She leaned over and kissed him warmly on the lips. "I love you, Jonas Willoughby. But Abigail is right. Until we forgive ourselves, we are never free to love anyone, not even ourselves. Later today I plan to go down to the vicarage and talk to Charles about forgiveness. I was hoping you would go with me."

He stared in disbelief. "I can't believe it. That's what I wanted to do—and have you go with me."

They stood up together. "Syd, I don't think I really wanted to find Conon. My commitment—my duty to Her Majesty and to my country—was to track him down and turn him in. But I tried to look at his children through your eyes and Abigail's, and I thought, 'Dear God, how can I do it?'"

From where they were, they heard Griselda say, "Come along, children. And, Gregor, take Abigail's arm."

As the door closed, Jonas resumed a familiar stance. Pensive. Distant. A handsome man with the sleeves of his shirt rolled up. His hands were flattened together, forefingers pressed to his lips, his eyes downcast. He seemed unaware that locks of his dark hair had fallen across his brow. Unaware of her.

"Jonas, I must go now. I'll be back."

He gave no indication of hearing her. "I felt all along that Abigail and Charles knew what was going on, but I never thought of Lucas. There's a loyalty to those of us with the Royal Navy."

"But you willingly blamed Abigail and Charles."

"They weren't wearing navy blue." His smile was forced. "Don't make me feel any worse. Lucas could have destroyed us all in that fire—because I couldn't see through the color blue."

Did she dare leave him? "Stop blaming yourself, Jonas."

"Abigail told me that the war between Conon and me had to end sometime. I didn't think it would end this way. If I had known he was dying, I would have asked Dr. Wallis to see him. But I wouldn't be able to meet Conon as a friend. Whichever path I took I would betray someone: Conon, the children, Her Majesty. And all through that struggle, something inside told me that Louise would want me to forgive Conon."

"Let God forgive you."

His eyes met hers, the hazy blue like drifting clouds.

"I have to go, Jonas. I wish you were going with me."

Outside, she fled down the hill to catch up with the others. When she arrived at the churchyard, strangers in town were arguing with Charles. "This grave must be dug up."

He towered above them. "I forbid any tampering of this grave site. This is church property."

"The man was an Irish terrorist. We need to identify him, make certain it is Conon O'Reilly—"

"Your terrorist is dead, gentlemen. You must take my word for it. You can gain nothing by digging up O'Reilly's body. Let the man rest in peace. He had so little peace in his lifetime."

Charles with his snow-white hair made an imposing figure towering above the strangers. His collar seemed to pinch his neck, an impressive velvet robe flapped at his ankles. They backed off.

But would they come back in the stealth of night? Sydney wondered.

Conon lay in an unmarked grave, beneath a crudely carved cross bearing the words *Rest in Peace.* Boris had helped the children nail the cross together and had himself painted the black letters against the wood. Clinging to Sydney's hand and her rag doll, Keeley stepped forward and placed a bouquet of hand-picked wildflowers on her father's grave. Many of the village folk who hunted him down had gathered to say farewell to Abigail's troubled Irish boy.

A slight breeze blew the vicar's hair. "Fly away, my son, like the dove," he intoned. "Conon O'Reilly, we must think of you as taking flight on the wings of a bird and finding shelter from your stormy life. Father, I believe he sought you in the end—"

As Charles spoke, the keening wail of bagpipes filled the air. Sydney glanced up and saw Jonas coming toward them in his Scottish kilts, coming steadily down the hill to the churchyard on those sturdy sun-tanned legs. The keening, lamenting wail of "Nearer, My God, to Thee" drifted out over the Cotswold Hills.

Sydney squeezed Keeley's shoulder and held tightly to Danny's hand. Suddenly Keeley pulled free and dropped her rag doll on the ground. She pointed toward the hills. "Papa. My papa."

Sympathy spread across the faces of the mourners, expressions that said "the child is grief stricken." But Sydney had seen her glancing off toward the golden hills. Surreptitiously, she looked and saw two men high on the hillside above the cemetery resting on saddled horses. She was certain that the thin young man on the hilltop was Conon O'Reilly. She glanced worriedly toward Abigail, but she stood serenely beside Griselda, a veil covering her face, her eyes fixed on the mound of dirt with its crudely shaped cross. Sydney glanced up again, but the sun blinded her. She saw nothing. No one. Not even a cloud of dust from horse and rider. A mirage? A phantom illusion? Her last desperate wish for life for Conon?

Her eyes strayed to Jonas. He met her gaze, unwavering. She knew in that instant that he had looked toward the hills as well. He showed no anger, no fury. He gave her a quick nod, and she realized that the strangers at the graveside had drifted away from the mourners and were racing toward their car. She and Jonas would share their secret. It was best this way, allowing the children and Abigail this time in the churchyard for a proper good-bye.

On Monday Sydney had her suitcases packed and sitting in one corner of the room with her laptop computer beside them. She and Jeff were leaving in the morning for Heathrow and the flight back home. She would come back someday. For now, the children at the manor would be safe with Abigail and Griselda and the newly hired staff.

With Jeff leaving, Blackstone and Rentley agreed to take on Sydney's long-term legal battle for custody of the O'Reilly children. But she braced herself for saying good-bye to Jonas. They would spend the afternoon together. Even now, he waited for her by the roses. As she ran down the steps, he plucked a vivid pink rose and handed it to her. Her garden! Her gardener!

"This is where it all began," she said. "The day I came back to Broadshire Manor, you were here pruning the roses."

"What did you think of me then?"

"That you were mighty handsome for a gardener. I was struck with how tall and strong you were. How tanned your skin was. How rugged you looked and yet how kind to Gregor you were. And when you looked at me over Gregor's head, your eyes were frosty blue."

"I wasn't doing a good job of pruning the roses. I kept watching you come up the hillside, looking poised and graceful." He pushed a stray strand of hair from her forehead. "I liked the way your hair was drawn back so I could see your face. I haven't been able to stop looking at you since you came. I think I knew the minute I saw you that you had walked into my life and I would fall in love again."

She remembered how their eyes had locked across the primroses and she blushed. "I'll miss you."

"Can we go for a walk?" he asked, catching her hand in his.

"Oh, Jonas, I promised the children—"

His smile faded. "All right. They can come as long as they give us space of our own."

They walked down toward the Windrush, the children stumbling and screaming ahead of them. "Will it always be like this, Sydney? Me competing for your time with the children?"

"Will you mind?"

"Not as long as you come back to me."

"Don't, Jonas. Don't make leaving any harder. You know we agreed to give each other space. Time to sort out our feelings."

"I already know that I want you to be part of my life. But without you here, life will be empty. Have you ever thought about how much you would give up for the one you love?"

"I always think about how much I would gain."

Off to their right, the steeple of St. Michael's towered with the trees. "You attended the service on Sunday," he said.

You know I did. We sat together on that hard narrow bench. We stared at the same stained-glass window. Heard the same music. Listened to the same message. But for most of that service Keeley wiggled beside me as I fixed my eyes on the baptismal font.

"Yes, I was there, Jonas."

"Do you remember what Reverend Rainford-Simms said?"

Her cheeks grew hot. She didn't remember one word of the sermon, only snatches of the parishioners rendering the morning reading from the Song of Songs. *I belong to my lover and his desire is for me.*

The sermon was on the sanctity of marriage, and she sat there filled with remorse that she had broken the vows of purity with Randolph Iverson. How could God or Jonas ever forgive her? How could she forgive herself for not waiting? Now the words of the sermon tumbled around in her thoughts as she realized how deeply she cared for Jonas Willoughby.

Jonas stopped on the trail and ran his fingers gently over her cheek. "I think Charles spoke on marriage for our sake. He has been the wise one, long ago setting me free to fall in love again. I was the one holding on to Louise's memory."

"I thought you let her go," she whispered.

"I did when we took that trip to Ireland. You have to believe me. You're the one who fills my thoughts now."

"But if you knew the truth about me—"

"The past? I guessed long ago that Randolph was more than a friend, Sydney. We both have regrets. Let's start over from this moment in time. Let's accept God's forgiveness for the past?" His eyes were pale blue this morning, full of love as he looked at her. "What do I have to do to get you to stay and marry me?"

You'd have to ask me.

"I can't stand the thought of you being on the other side of the pond. On Sunday, Charles quoted Solomon, saying that water can't quench love, nor rivers wash it away. Don't put an ocean between us. Having you here in England is what matters to me. I want to spend my life with you."

As they stood by the Windrush, the children ran circles around them. Jonas dug into his pocket for some money. "Gregor, Sydney and I have some serious business to discuss. I want you to take the children and buy some sweets at Veronica's Tea Shoppe."

335

Gregor's lower lip trembled. He scowled at the younger children. "Come on," he ordered.

"Gregor—son," Jonas called.

Gregor caught his balance, dug in with his toes turned in, his eyes cast down. "Yes."

"Whatever Sydney and I decide, Gregor, you will be part of our plans. We'll include you in any plans we make."

"You won't make me go to Gordonstoun right away?"

"Not until you're ready."

"What about Keeley and Danny?"

"Them too."

"And the others—Tesa and Philip and Yasmin?"

"Abigail is making long-term arrangements for them when the National Trust comes in to restore the property. But we won't let them go unless it's a happy place."

He took Sydney's hand as the children ran off. "I'll ring you every week. Every day."

"Try e-mail," she said. "It's less expensive. Save your money for my ring."

"You'll have your ring. The biggest one I can find. But an ocean will separate us, Sydney—your country and mine. That's what worries me."

Beside them they heard the powerful rush of the river sweeping under the bridge and crashing over the rocks, and then flowing gently on. "There's no ocean here, Jonas. Just the River Windrush. And there's a bridge across that. We can bridge our differences, but we still need some time."

"What about your place on Lake Washington?"

"It's too big for one person. It was too big when my parents were alive, but it was home. I grew up in its rambling rooms, but I could let it go if I moved back here. But my retreat by the river—I can't let that go. I want to take the children back there every summer—or maybe at Christmas some time. Gregor will especially love it."

"I won't always be free to go with you."

336

"I know. You'll be at sea. But sometimes you can go with us. I want you to know and love that place as I do."

"And your job at Barrington Enterprises?"

"I worked out my options in case you invited me back. It's too soon for me to quit. We've just won the first phase of our bid on the carriers. They won't even be launched until 2012."

"I can't wait that long—I'd be an old man."

She laughed. "Just a few years older than you are now. But I'm talking about three months to make arrangements at home."

"And what do you have in that calculating mind of yours?"

"I'll keep the controlling interest in the company. I'll appoint someone else as CEO. In other words, I'll turn over the day-to-day operations."

"To Randolph Iverson?"

"He's the best man for the job. He wanted it in the first place. But I'll stay on as chairman of the board."

"What a business head you are. But how do you plan to juggle being a wife and mother with running Barrington Enterprises?"

"I'll plan quarterly board meetings—I'll fly over for those. And there's nothing to stop me from calling the board of directors to the Jarrow Shipyard. That would be convenient for me." She grinned. "I've had weeks working these details out in my mind in case you got around to asking me to marry you."

"Will you ever sell out—after you marry me?"

"Someday. I've had offers to merge. But I'm not stepping down until the carriers are commissioned. If you're going to be on board, I want them to be the best construction ever."

"They will be," he said, slipping his arm around her.

"I don't want to sell Barrington until we're the top defense company ever, and even then, I'll keep a controlling interest and remain a stockholder. Dad won't know, but if he did, I'd want him to be proud of the job I did and the choice I make when it's time to merge. Even when I sell, I'll only do so if the buyout keeps me on the board of directors for five or ten years."

"What about that option on a shipyard in Italy?"

"I'm still negotiating. I think it's to our advantage to have several plants here in Europe."

"You amaze me. But what guarantee do I have that you'll come back and marry me?"

They had been walking along the Windrush. She stopped and faced him. Standing on tiptoe she threw her arms around her Englishman's neck and hugged him.

"Is this guarantee enough?" she asked. She was laughing up at him, her lips parted, her eyes surely dancing. He put his arms tightly around her and drew her closer. She was still smiling, laughing as his lips came down hard on hers.

Epilogue

Abigail and the Admiral sat in the garden watching the mist rise as dawn spread its copper wings over the Cotswold Hills. Autumn had come to Stow-on-the-Woodland, brushing the land with patches of amber and jonquil yellow. The primrose bushes had been pruned back, and the ground lay russet like winter apples. Harvest dominated the countryside with farmers and combines already at work. Everything had changed with the season, everything but the constancy of the hills.

Abigail was grateful to see another sunrise when sunset was so close for both of them. Long after she and the Admiral were gone, strangers would come to sit in this quaint gazebo sheltered from the winds and dampness and find comfort, as she did, looking down on the meandering river and across at the hills bathed in coppery autumn hues. Their early morning ritual was always the same now. Griselda bundled them up in sturdy warm jackets and left them outside for an hour with lap robes snug around their legs to ward off the biting chill. Then she would hustle them inside to the drawing room where she served them tea and crumpets by the fire.

These autumn days brought color to the Admiral's cheeks, but Dr. Wallis fussed about Abigail sitting in the wind, fearing she would get her death of chill. She told him a woman on borrowed time needed the scent of fresh air and the sun on her face.

From her chair, she could see the ongoing facelift for St. Michael's. Inside the manor, the east and south wings resonated with hammering and shouting men as the National Trust began its restorations on Broadshire Manor. They had agreed to let Santos work in the gallery each morning to restore the vivid beauty to ancient works of art, one painting at a time.

Abigail folded her hands over the letter from Charles Rainford-Simms and thought of him in the North country, content with a small plot of land of his own. When she wrote again, she would tell him about the new cleric at St. Michael's, the young man in his first pastorate, vibrant with ideas for enlarging his congregation. She would not mention the lively beat of the music or the cleverly worded sermons that parishioners forgot as they reached the door. But she would tell Charles about the autumn colors that covered the hillsides when Griselda walked down to put flowers on Louise's and Conon's graves. He always asked about the children—and she had told him they were back at the primary school.

She would miss her children, yet she had come to life's full circle—the hidden children of wars no longer came to her, but she had memories of dozens of boys and girls tucked away in her heart. A lifetime of treasures. Charles would not ask, but she knew he would wonder whether she had found the courage to tell Jonas the truth. Her silence still taunted her. She regretted Jonas not knowing that he was her son, and it saddened her that the girl she would have chosen for Jonas herself had gone back to her powerful position at Barrington Enterprises. But with Charles, she confided her sadness about the Admiral's continued decline, his memory wheel clogged more and more in the past.

But this is a good day, Abigail thought. *Tobias is fresh and alert.*

She sighed and the Admiral rallied from his first nap of the day. He sent a swift glance her way, pleasure filling his face.

"My dear, is something wrong?"

"Nothing," she told him.

"What happened to that young woman who used to visit me?"

She had told him many times, but patiently she said, "Sydney went back to America. Remember?"

"I miss her. I thought Jonas really fancied her."

"He did."

He mulled that over, and she was certain that he had slipped back to the past, to the glory days of ships and sailing, back even to the day he was knighted by the Queen. He remembered that sometimes with great pride and his eyes bright with memory.

Instead, he surprised her, saying, "I've worried about you, Abby. Where have you been?"

She patted his hand. "I told you yesterday." She regretted the sharpness in her tone and added, "I was ill, James, for a long time. But I'm better now."

"I thought you were gone—without Jonas knowing the truth."

Her heart fluttered. Skipped a bit. "The truth, Tobias?"

He covered her hand with his own. "I did love you. But I could not leave Helen. She needed me. I needed her."

Abigail nodded—allowing her hand to remain in his. "After she died, Tobias, I thought the two of us—"

"That would have been wrong, dear Abby. Jonas needed the memory of his mother. Abigail, what a mess I made of our lives."

He closed his eyes and forced himself back to the moment. "My memory is not as good as it used to be. Where was I?"

"You were talking about Helen."

"No. No, I was talking about us. I never admitted to you that I knew about Jonas. I wanted nothing to mar my reputation or ruin my career."

She leaned against him. "I know, James. I've always known."

"Have you ever told Jonas?"

341

"No, there's no need to tell him now."

"But I know," Jonas said, coming out to the garden to join them. "I know that you are my mother."

She turned and watched her son coming toward her. *He knows. He knows he is my son.* She felt strength in his height, in his unwavering gaze. He stood with his hand resting on the rail of the gazebo. She longed to stand up and hug him— to dance with him. To tell him she had loved him forever.

"How?" she whispered, staring up at him. "How did you know?"

"Sitting with my father, night after night. The hours between midnight and dawn are long. He was always calling for you, and I began to wonder why."

"I'm so sorry."

"No, don't be. When I told Sydney that I knew, she told me I was lucky. I had two mothers who loved me. One who made a great sacrifice for me."

He crossed the lawn that separated them and put his hand firmly on her shoulder. "I've known for a long time that you've loved my father. You've sacrificed your life for him. Perhaps that is one of the reasons I was so angry at him."

"I wanted to be here in the manor so I could be close to you—to watch you grow up—to be here whenever you came home."

"You've always been here for me, Abigail."

"Oh, Jonas. At last I can shout it to the world that you are my son. I don't have to go on pretending."

His face clouded. "We can't make a grand announcement. Stow-on-the-Woodland is a small town. And my uncle would never understand. I don't want to hurt him. The Willoughbys are a proud people. And Dad's reputation— his long Navy career—would be ruined. Can we go on as we've been?"

Silently? Robbed always of motherhood? She choked up. So close, but she was still to bear the secret to her grave. Her voice trembled. "Yes, if that's what you want. Yes."

342

"I can never tell the truth outside the manor—for the sake and reputation of the Willoughby family. I'll tell my commanding officer. I am obligated to do so."

"Oh, Jonas, it could ruin you ever reaching the Admiralty."

"We'll let Captain McIntyre decide how it will affect my career." He leaned down and kissed the top of her head. "Abigail, you've been a good mother. I love you for that."

She held his hand against her cheek, kissed the palm, tears washing down her cheeks. "What will you do now?"

"I'm going back to sea soon. You and Dad will stay on here at the manor for as long as you want. Or I can move you to a residence where you will be well cared for. But Sydney will not hear of this—"

"We thought you would marry Sydney. And then she left."

"She's coming back, and she's determined to arrange for even more help for Griselda so you can live out your lives here."

"And the children?"

"You already know we've found homes for three of them. Tesa to distant relatives. And Blackstone and Rentley found a temporary home for Philip and Yasmin with an American couple in the northern Cotswolds."

Her throat constricted. She had never sent any of her children away willingly. "Will they treat them kindly?"

"Blackstone thinks so. The father is a photojournalist— the mother a biologist. They have a little girl of their own and an adopted son."

"But it's only a temporary home?"

He smiled. "Blackstone knows the family personally. He says once they see Yasmin and Philip, they'll never let them go. But we won't send them until after Christmas. You'll want that last Christmas together."

"You won't separate Danny and Keeley?"

"No. Sydney would not hear of it. Between the American embassy going to bat for her and the barrister in London making special arrangements, Sydney will be free to take them to America next summer."

"I was so hoping—"

"She's coming back, Abigail," he said with a grin. "I've asked her to marry me. Those trips to America with the children will be holiday times."

"And Gregor?" She asked with reprimand in her voice and the dreaded fear that Gregor would be lost and alone.

"Poor Sydney," he said, smiling even more. "When she gets me, she gets all three children. . . . I think that will make you and Dad grandparents. Will you mind?"

Abigail tightened her grip over the Admiral's frail hand, her own vein-riddled one tissue-thin. "We will be very proud."

"From now on, Abby, I will think of you as my mother. But things must go on the way they have always been. You will always be the friend of the family. You do understand, don't you?"

"I didn't even deserve this much."

"But you do," the Admiral said. "You have deserved so much more than I ever gave you. Jonas—Abigail—can you forgive an old man his sin and selfishness? I have denied you both for so long."

Jonas—proud man that he was—embraced his father. "We'll go on from here, Dad. Next weekend, I will bring you a surprise, Abby. A celebration of motherhood and how much you mean to me."

"A surprise for me? Not the children?"

"They will enjoy my surprise as well. So will you, Dad."

He bent low and whispered gently in his mother's ear, "Thank you for all you've done for me. I love you, Abby. I'll see you both next weekend."

"Don't forget my surprise."

She watched this son of hers go in a brisk stride, confident in his own future, and, as he always did, he went away with her heart. She heard the engine of his car turn over and then he was racing toward London. Jonas Willoughby, her son.

"Who was that young man who just drove away?" the Admiral asked. "He's wearing the uniform of the Royal Navy."

"He's your son, Tobias. He followed in your footsteps."

He frowned, perplexed, grasping at the threads of memory. "You mean that little boy has grown up? I thought he was still away at Gordonstoun."

"That was many years ago."

"I'd forgotten. I'm glad he's with the Navy. He seems like a nice young man. Is he with the Admiralty?"

"Not yet. But he is a wonderful young man. He's your son. How could he be anything less?"

"If that's my son, I should have told him how proud I am of him. How much I love him. I wonder if he knows?"

"Why don't you tell him the next time he comes?"

The Admiral dozed again and moments later awakened to the present again, looking cheerful and alert. He threw aside his lap robe. "Abby, I am cold. I think we should go inside."

"Griselda will be along shortly to get us."

His old mischief curled the corners of his mouth into a smile. "But I'm inviting you to have tea with me, my lady."

He stood unsteadily and reached out his hand to her. They linked arms for balance and began the incredible task of climbing the stone steps. Abigail had forgotten how tall Tobias was; he was so much like his charming son, his hair still raven black with only fringes of gray at the temple. He gave her his rakish grin, and those once slaty blue eyes, faded now, held a special glint in them for her.

Even his voice filled with laughter when he said, "Tomorrow I might not remember you, but today, my dear Abby, I do."

"Today is all that matters, Sir James."

And together they went up the last few steps and into the manor where the Admiral would have tea with his lady.

Jonas glanced at his watch. In another three hours he would hear Sydney's voice again and be able to tell her how much he loved her. She was flying high above the ocean, every second bringing her closer to the landing at Heathrow.

As he strode briskly toward the parking zone at Northwood, Captain McIntyre stopped him. "I wanted to catch you, Commander. So you're on your way to the airport already? And you're wearing your uniform to meet your girl?"

"Yes, she's never seen me in it, sir. I'm stopping off at the Hollinsworths' en route."

"Checking up on Jock again? He's had a rough recovery. But thanks to you, Commander, he's still alive."

"We'll both be flying again soon."

"You've earned wearing those wings again. I'll miss working with you at Northwood. Your stubbornness did your friend a favor. The disaster investigation would have delayed our search for him for months if you hadn't insisted that he wasn't on board."

"It still took too long before we found him."

"Tell Mr. Hollinsworth that they spotted Lucas Sullivan in Belfast. It's only a matter of time before he's in custody. According to his own men, he planned to commandeer that Learjet from the day Jock visited you in Stow-on-the-Woodland."

"Yes, I already told Jock. But no word on Conon?"

McIntyre's face clouded. "We've put off telling you. Sullivan dumped Conon O'Reilly off on his father-in-law's farm. Conon's in-laws took him in and arranged medical care for him."

"But Sean Callahan despises his son-in-law."

"True," McIntyre said philosophically. "But his wife was more merciful. She refused to turn the father of her grandchildren away again."

"That didn't bother Callahan before."

"Apparently a talk with the local priest persuaded him otherwise."

Jonas saw Sydney's dreams of mothering Keeley and Danny slipping from them. "Should I tell my fiancée and Abigail Broderick that he's been found alive?"

The captain rubbed his jaw with vigor. "It would only raise false hopes. We have a watch on the farm to keep abreast of the comings and goings. But the British won't even press charges against Conon. It's too late for that. When the lad reached his father-in-law's farm, his gunshot wounds were too infected. Conon O'Reilly won't live long. He's in and out of a coma—wouldn't even recognize his children if you took them to him. Best they remember him the way they last saw him."

Jonas shook the hand extended to him. "Then I'll be off, sir."

"Commander, I'm looking forward to meeting that fiancée of yours."

He patted the jewel box in his pocket. "So am I, sir."

After a brief visit with the Hollinsworths, Jonas reached Heathrow early and paced back and forth in the terminal until the announcement came that Sydney's plane was on the runway. His spine stiffened. He had an attack of the jitters. What if she changed her mind when she saw him? What if distance had changed them both?

The seconds ticked away. The minutes. Every welcoming speech he had prepared vanished. He had forgotten to pick up the flowers he had ordered that morning. He brushed his jacket with his hand for the third time. Checked his watch. Took his cap off and put it back on. She wanted to see him in full uniform.

His forehead felt damp, his collar too tight.

The passengers coming off the plane were detained behind a rope barrier while airline personnel consulted a passenger list.

He saw Sydney now and his fears vanished. Every fiber in his body came alive with longing to hold her. To not let her go.

Now she saw him and her smile matched his. She was more lovely than he remembered.

"Jonas."

He called back, "I thought your plane would never get here."

"We're four minutes early."

They were doing gymnastics trying to keep their eye on each other. He stretched, looking beyond the burly man in front of her. "I didn't think you'd be back so soon. My calendar is worn thin with counting the days."

She stood on tiptoe and steadied herself, grabbing the man's arm. "I didn't want to wait three months to see you again."

"Jump over the rope, sweetheart; I'll catch you!" he called.

"I'll toss her over," the burly man offered.

She laughed, her laugh as bubbly as the Windrush. "I love you, Commander Willoughby."

"I love you more, Sydney Barrington."

The people around them chuckled.

"I forgot the roses," he said.

"It doesn't matter. We have a lifetime to gather flowers."

The rope blocking their way was removed. The weary travelers pushed forward and then Jonas called out, "Barrel your way through, sweetheart. I love you. I'm waiting."

Suddenly the surging crowd fanned back, making a path for love. Jonas opened his arms wide as Sydney came running to him. He swept her up into his arms and whispered in her ear, "I love you, Sydney. And I will never, never let an ocean separate us again."

Doris Elaine Fell followed a multifaceted career as teacher, missionary nurse, and freelance editor and author. Her writing credits include more than fifteen books and numerous articles. She writes from her home in Huntington Beach, California.